Welcome dear new vegans and long-time vegans,

may you find this journal a great tool to support your journey

of positive change, and may this also be a healing process for

maintaining well-being in a non-vegan world.

Remember vegan is love, keep your love burning in your heart,

it will spread and touch others...

Your seeds of compassion will be sewn...

Love

Kasarah Vegan xx

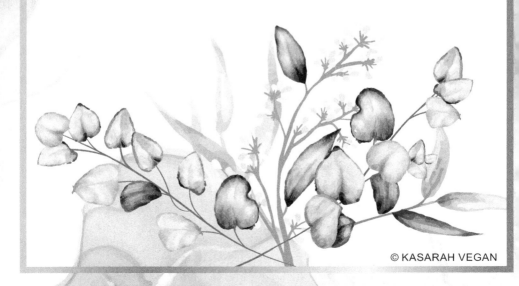

CONTENTS

MY PRIORITIES

My priority reasons for becoming, or already being vegan.

What are your reasons ?

_____
_____
_____
_____
_____
_____
_____
_____
_____
_____

What has encouraged you take this step ?

_____
_____
_____
_____
_____
_____
_____
_____
_____
_____
_____

MY PRIORITIES

My priority reasons for becoming, or already being vegan.

What has influenced you?

_____
_____
_____
_____
_____
_____
_____
_____
_____
_____

What maintains you, or what do you think will maintain your journey?

_____
_____
_____
_____
_____
_____
_____
_____
_____
_____
_____

CHALLENGES

My biggest challenges I need to face with becoming
(or being) vegan in a predominantly non-vegan world:

_____

_____

_____

_____

_____

_____

_____

_____

_____

_____

_____

_____

_____

_____

_____

_____

_____

_____

_____

_____

_____

_____

_____

_____

_____

_____

_____

_____

CHALLENGES

My biggest challenges I need to face with becoming
(or being) vegan in a predominantly non-vegan world:

_____

_____

_____

_____

_____

_____

_____

_____

_____

_____

_____

_____

_____

_____

_____

_____

_____

_____

_____

_____

_____

_____

_____

_____

_____

VEGAN NUTRITION QUICK GUIDE

I am not a nutritionist, dietician or doctor but I have a qualification in regard to supplements and the body-systems and a general interest in food, supplements and health.

Before starting any new vitamins or supplements, do check with a medical health or diet specialist; especially if you have any medical conditions and if you take medications and/or supplements already.

Protein — Daily amounts required is around 50 grams for adults, likely to be higher for athletes.

Calcium — Daily amount required is around 700mg for both male and female adults.

Iron — Daily amount required is around 8.7mg for men and women over 50yrs, younger women will require around 14-15mg per day.

VEGAN SUPPLEMENTATION

Vitamin C — Daily amount required around 40mg is required as a minimum, 1000mg maximum generally.

It can be obtained easily through a balanced wholefood diet.

Generally most vitamins, minerals can be obtained through eating a wholefood vegan diet, but it is best to take Algae supplements for Omega 3 EPA and DHA, Vitamin B12 and Vitamin D for maintaining a healthy immune system.

Vitamin D — How it supports the body: Supports health of bones and teeth, immune system, helps with calcium absorption.

This is now being more recognised in regard to keeping a healthy immune system. Depending where in the world you live or the tone of your skin, will depend on how much or little vitamin D you will obtain from the sun and absorb in regard to your life-style. Generally vitamin D is safe to take but anyone taking 3000mg or above will need to either speak with a doctor who has knowledge of vitamin D or a nutritionist with this knowledge due to vitamin D being a fat soluble vitamin that can build up in the liver and potentially cause toxicity if doses taken are too large.

VEGAN SUPPLEMENTATION

B12 (Cobalamin) — How it supports the body: Supports nerve health, boosts mood and energy levels.

A vitamin of the earth but it is no longer available from the soil naturally so it usually synthetically made and added into foods such as breakfast cereals, yeast extract or nutritional yeast flakes. Supplements can be used on their own or within a vitamin B complex supplement. Vitamin B12 is not always absorbed by people with specific health conditions. Recommended dose is around 1000-2000 mg per day.

Vitamin C — How it supports the body: Collagen in the skin and body, immune system support (also works well with zinc) It can be obtained from a number of fruits and vegetables, especially bell peppers, guavas, broccoli, kiwis which are high in Vitamin C.

VEGAN SUPPLEMENTATION

Omega 3 — How it supports the body: Maintains a balanced health for the heart, blood pressure, blood cholesterol, brain function and eye-sight.

Guidance can vary on the dosage per day, which is usually suggested to be 200mg and higher, sometimes as high as 2000mg for people with health conditions who have been advised to take higher amounts. Omega 3 with EPA and DHA is said to be important. Algae supplements are available for EPA and DHA. Walnuts and flaxseeds are good source of ALA.

Selenium — How it supports the body: Strengthens the immune system, muscle health, good eyesight, maintains skin elasticity, and is a powerful anti-oxidant.

If you like Brazil nuts, then a daily 2 or 3 of these should provide the selenium required.

VEGAN SUPPLEMENTATION

Iodine – How it supports the body: Helps balance metabolism, supports mental function and prevents fatigue. (May interact with thyroid medications – must check with medical professional before taking, as it may be advised not to take Iodine).

For a multi-vitamin that covers most of the above (apart from omega 3, and low strength vitamin D) The Vegan Society sell chewable vitamins called Veg1. There are other brands of vegan multi-vitamins to choose from too.

VEGAN SUPPLEMENTATION

Make some efforts to have a little time to keep up to date with research, as new discoveries and better understanding of the body, food, nutrients and supplements are being developed and advanced regularly.

I find Dr Greger's Nutrition Facts website to be of great use and very interesting. Try to eat as many wholefoods as possible, and reduce intake of simple carbs, refined sugary and processed foods.

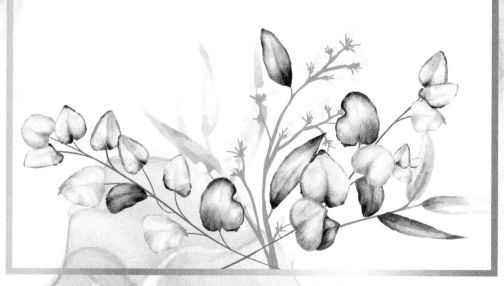

MEAL PLANNING

My 7 day breakfast options

It is ok to have the same, but a variety of ideas may suit you too

Day 1:
_____

_____

_____

_____

_____

Day 2:
_____

_____

_____

_____

_____

Day 3:
_____

_____

_____

_____

_____

Day 4: _____
_____

_____
_____
_____
_____

Day 5: _____
_____

_____
_____
_____
_____

Day 6: _____
_____

_____
_____
_____
_____

Day 7: _____
_____

_____
_____
_____
_____

MEAL PLANNING

My 7 day lunch options for at Work or at home

Day 1:

_____
_____
_____
_____
_____
_____

Day 2:

_____
_____
_____
_____
_____
_____

Day 3:

_____
_____
_____
_____
_____

Day 4:

_____

_____

_____

_____

_____

Day 5:

_____

_____

_____

_____

_____

Day 6:

_____

_____

_____

_____

_____

Day 7:

_____

_____

_____

_____

_____

MEAL PLANNING

My 7 day dinner options for at Work or at home

Day 1:

_____
_____
_____
_____
_____
_____

Day 2:

_____
_____
_____
_____
_____
_____

Day 3:

_____
_____
_____
_____
_____

Day 4: _____

_____

_____

_____

_____

Day 5: _____

_____

_____

_____

_____

Day 6: _____

_____

_____

_____

_____

Day 7: _____

_____

_____

_____

_____

MEAL PLANNING

My snack options for at Work or at home

Day 1:
_____
_____
_____
_____
_____

Day 2:
_____
_____
_____
_____
_____

Day 3:
_____
_____
_____
_____
_____

Day 4: _____
_____
_____
_____
_____

Day 5: _____
_____
_____
_____
_____

Day 6: _____
_____
_____
_____
_____

Day 7: _____
_____
_____
_____
_____

MEAL PLANNING

My dessert options for at Work or at home

Day 1:
_____
_____
_____
_____
_____
_____

Day 2:
_____
_____
_____
_____
_____
_____

Day 3:
_____
_____
_____
_____
_____

Day 4: _____

_____

_____

_____

_____

Day 5: _____

_____

_____

_____

_____

Day 6: _____

_____

_____

_____

_____

Day 7: _____

_____

_____

_____

_____

MY DAILY VEGAN

Day 1: _____

How did my day go?

_____
_____
_____
_____
_____
_____
_____
_____
_____
_____
_____
_____
_____
_____
_____
_____
_____
_____
_____
_____
_____
_____
_____
_____
_____
_____

Has my food intake been sufficient in:

Protein ☐   Calcium ☐   Iron ☐   Omega 3 ☐   Vitamin C ☐   Fibre ☐

Notes

How has my mood been today?

_____
_____
_____
_____
_____
_____

Is there anything I would do differently the following days?
(This could be in regard to your food intake, your discussions about veganism with others, dealing with difficult scenarios with non-vegans etc)

_____
_____
_____
_____
_____
_____
_____

MY DAILY VEGAN DIARY

Day 2: _____

How did my day go?

_____
_____
_____
_____
_____
_____
_____
_____
_____
_____
_____
_____
_____
_____
_____
_____
_____
_____
_____
_____
_____
_____
_____
_____
_____
_____
_____
_____

Has my food intake been sufficient in:

Protein ☐   Calcium ☐   Iron ☐   Omega 3 ☐   Vitamin C ☐   Fibre ☐

Notes

How has my mood been today?

Is there anything I would do differently the following days?

(This could be in regard to your food intake, your discussions about veganism with others, dealing with difficult scenarios with non-vegans etc)

MY DAILY VEGAN DIARY

Day 3: _____

How did my day go?

_____
_____
_____
_____
_____
_____
_____
_____
_____
_____
_____
_____
_____
_____
_____
_____
_____
_____
_____
_____
_____
_____
_____
_____
_____
_____
_____
_____

Has my food intake been sufficient in:

Protein ☐   Calcium ☐   Iron ☐   Omega 3 ☐   Vitamin C ☐   Fibre ☐

Notes

How has my mood been today?

_____
_____
_____
_____
_____
_____

Is there anything I would do differently the following days?
(This could be in regard to your food intake, your discussions about veganism with others, dealing with difficult scenarios with non-vegans etc)

_____
_____
_____
_____
_____
_____
_____

MY DAILY VEGAN DIARY

Day 4:

How did my day go?

_____
_____
_____
_____
_____
_____
_____
_____
_____
_____
_____
_____
_____
_____
_____
_____
_____
_____
_____
_____
_____
_____
_____
_____
_____

Has my food intake been sufficient in:

Protein ☐   Calcium ☐   Iron ☐   Omega 3 ☐   Vitamin C ☐   Fibre ☐

Notes

How has my mood been today?

_____
_____
_____
_____
_____
_____

Is there anything I would do differently the following days?
(This could be in regard to your food intake, your discussions about veganism with others, dealing with difficult scenarios with non-vegans etc)

_____
_____
_____
_____
_____
_____
_____

MY DAILY VEGAN DIARY

Day 5: _____

How did my day go?

_____
_____
_____
_____
_____
_____
_____
_____
_____
_____
_____
_____
_____
_____
_____
_____
_____
_____
_____
_____
_____
_____
_____
_____
_____
_____
_____
_____
_____

Has my food intake been sufficient in:

Protein ☐   Calcium ☐   Iron ☐   Omega 3 ☐   Vitamin C ☐   Fibre ☐

Notes

How has my mood been today?

_____

_____

_____

_____

_____

_____

Is there anything I would do differently the following days?

(This could be in regard to your food intake, your discussions about veganism with others, dealing with difficult scenarios with non-vegans etc)

_____

_____

_____

_____

_____

_____

_____

MY DAILY VEGAN DIARY

Day 6: _____

How did my day go?

_____
_____
_____
_____
_____
_____
_____
_____
_____
_____
_____
_____
_____
_____
_____
_____
_____
_____
_____
_____
_____
_____
_____
_____
_____
_____
_____

Has my food intake been sufficient in:

Protein ☐   Calcium ☐   Iron ☐   Omega 3 ☐   Vitamin C ☐   Fibre ☐

Notes

How has my mood been today?

_____

_____

_____

_____

_____

Is there anything I would do differently the following days?

(This could be in regard to your food intake, your discussions about

veganism with others, dealing with difficult scenarios with non-vegans

etc)

_____

_____

_____

_____

_____

_____

MY DAILY VEGAN DIARY

Day 7: _____

How did my day go?

_____
_____
_____
_____
_____
_____
_____
_____
_____
_____
_____
_____
_____
_____
_____
_____
_____
_____
_____
_____
_____
_____
_____
_____
_____
_____
_____
_____

Has my food intake been sufficient in:

Protein ☐   Calcium ☐   Iron ☐   Omega 3 ☐   Vitamin C ☐   Fibre ☐

Notes

How has my mood been today?

_____
_____
_____
_____
_____
_____

Is there anything I would do differently the following days?
(This could be in regard to your food intake, your discussions about
veganism with others, dealing with difficult scenarios with non-vegans
etc)

_____
_____
_____
_____
_____
_____
_____

MY DAILY VEGAN DIARY

Day 8: _____

How did my day go?

_____
_____
_____
_____
_____
_____
_____
_____
_____
_____
_____
_____
_____
_____
_____
_____
_____
_____
_____
_____
_____
_____
_____
_____
_____
_____
_____
_____

Has my food intake been sufficient in:

Protein ☐   Calcium ☐   Iron ☐   Omega 3 ☐   Vitamin C ☐   Fibre ☐

Notes

How has my mood been today?

_____

_____

_____

_____

_____

_____

Is there anything I would do differently the following days?

(This could be in regard to your food intake, your discussions about

veganism with others, dealing with difficult scenarios with non-vegans

etc)

_____

_____

_____

_____

_____

_____

_____

MY DAILY VEGAN DIARY

Day 9: _____

How did my day go?

_____
_____
_____
_____
_____
_____
_____
_____
_____
_____
_____
_____
_____
_____
_____
_____
_____
_____
_____
_____
_____
_____
_____
_____
_____
_____
_____
_____

Has my food intake been sufficient in:

Protein ☐   Calcium ☐   Iron ☐   Omega 3 ☐   Vitamin C ☐   Fibre ☐

Notes

How has my mood been today?

_____

_____

_____

_____

_____

_____

Is there anything I would do differently the following days?

(This could be in regard to your food intake, your discussions about veganism with others, dealing with difficult scenarios with non-vegans etc)

_____

_____

_____

_____

_____

_____

_____

MY DAILY VEGAN DIARY

Day 10:

How did my day go?

_____
_____
_____
_____
_____
_____
_____
_____
_____
_____
_____
_____
_____
_____
_____
_____
_____
_____
_____
_____
_____
_____
_____
_____
_____
_____
_____
_____
_____
_____

Has my food intake been sufficient in:

Protein ☐   Calcium ☐   Iron ☐   Omega 3 ☐   Vitamin C ☐   Fibre ☐

Notes

How has my mood been today?

Is there anything I would do differently the following days?

(This could be in regard to your food intake, your discussions about

veganism with others, dealing with difficult scenarios with non-vegans

etc)

MY DAILY VEGAN DIARY

Day 11: _____

How did my day go?

_____
_____
_____
_____
_____
_____
_____
_____
_____
_____
_____
_____
_____
_____
_____
_____
_____
_____
_____
_____
_____
_____
_____
_____
_____
_____
_____

Has my food intake been sufficient in:

Protein ☐   Calcium ☐   Iron ☐   Omega 3 ☐   Vitamin C ☐   Fibre ☐

Notes

How has my mood been today?

_____

_____

_____

_____

_____

_____

Is there anything I would do differently the following days?

(This could be in regard to your food intake, your discussions about veganism with others, dealing with difficult scenarios with non-vegans etc)

_____

_____

_____

_____

_____

_____

_____

MY DAILY VEGAN DIARY

Day 12: _____

How did my day go?

_____
_____
_____
_____
_____
_____
_____
_____
_____
_____
_____
_____
_____
_____
_____
_____
_____
_____
_____
_____
_____
_____
_____
_____
_____
_____
_____
_____

Has my food intake been sufficient in:

Protein ☐   Calcium ☐   Iron ☐   Omega 3 ☐   Vitamin C ☐   Fibre ☐

Notes

How has my mood been today?

_____

_____

_____

_____

_____

_____

Is there anything I would do differently the following days?

(This could be in regard to your food intake, your discussions about

veganism with others, dealing with difficult scenarios with non-vegans

etc)

_____

_____

_____

_____

_____

_____

_____

MY DAILY VEGAN DIARY

Day 13. _____

How did my day go?

_____
_____
_____
_____
_____
_____
_____
_____
_____
_____
_____
_____
_____
_____
_____
_____
_____
_____
_____
_____
_____
_____
_____
_____
_____
_____
_____
_____
_____

Has my food intake been sufficient in:

Protein ☐   Calcium ☐   Iron ☐   Omega 3 ☐   Vitamin C ☐   Fibre ☐

Notes

How has my mood been today?

Is there anything I would do differently the following days?
(This could be in regard to your food intake, your discussions about veganism with others, dealing with difficult scenarios with non-vegans etc)

MY DAILY VEGAN DIARY

Day 14: _____

How did my day go?

_____
_____
_____
_____
_____
_____
_____
_____
_____
_____
_____
_____
_____
_____
_____
_____
_____
_____
_____
_____
_____
_____
_____
_____
_____
_____
_____

Has my food intake been sufficient in:

Protein ☐   Calcium ☐   Iron ☐   Omega 3 ☐   Vitamin C ☐   Fibre ☐

Notes

How has my mood been today?

_____

_____

_____

_____

_____

_____

Is there anything I would do differently the following days?
(This could be in regard to your food intake, your discussions about veganism with others, dealing with difficult scenarios with non-vegans etc)

_____

_____

_____

_____

_____

_____

_____

MY DAILY VEGAN DIARY

Day 15. _____

How did my day go?

_____
_____
_____
_____
_____
_____
_____
_____
_____
_____
_____
_____
_____
_____
_____
_____
_____
_____
_____
_____
_____
_____
_____
_____
_____
_____
_____
_____
_____
_____

Has my food intake been sufficient in:

Protein ☐   Calcium ☐   Iron ☐   Omega 3 ☐   Vitamin C ☐   Fibre ☐

Notes

How has my mood been today?

_____

_____

_____

_____

_____

_____

Is there anything I would do differently the following days?

(This could be in regard to your food intake, your discussions about

veganism with others, dealing with difficult scenarios with non-vegans

etc)

_____

_____

_____

_____

_____

_____

_____

MY DAILY VEGAN DIARY

Day 16.

How did my day go?

_____
_____
_____
_____
_____
_____
_____
_____
_____
_____
_____
_____
_____
_____
_____
_____
_____
_____
_____
_____
_____
_____
_____
_____
_____
_____

Has my food intake been sufficient in:

Protein ☐   Calcium ☐   Iron ☐   Omega 3 ☐   Vitamin C ☐   Fibre ☐

Notes

How has my mood been today?

_____
_____
_____
_____
_____
_____

Is there anything I would do differently the following days?
(This could be in regard to your food intake, your discussions about veganism with others, dealing with difficult scenarios with non-vegans etc)

_____
_____
_____
_____
_____
_____
_____

MY DAILY VEGAN DIARY

Day 17.

How did my day go?

_____
_____
_____
_____
_____
_____
_____
_____
_____
_____
_____
_____
_____
_____
_____
_____
_____
_____
_____
_____
_____
_____
_____
_____
_____
_____
_____
_____

Has my food intake been sufficient in:

Protein ☐   Calcium ☐   Iron ☐   Omega 3 ☐   Vitamin C ☐   Fibre ☐

Notes

How has my mood been today?

Is there anything I would do differently the following days?
(This could be in regard to your food intake, your discussions about veganism with others, dealing with difficult scenarios with non-vegans etc)

MY DAILY VEGAN DIARY

Day 18: _____

How did my day go?

_____
_____
_____
_____
_____
_____
_____
_____
_____
_____
_____
_____
_____
_____
_____
_____
_____
_____
_____
_____
_____
_____
_____
_____
_____
_____
_____
_____
_____
_____
_____
_____

Has my food intake been sufficient in:

Protein ☐   Calcium ☐   Iron ☐   Omega 3 ☐   Vitamin C ☐   Fibre ☐

Notes

How has my mood been today?

_____

_____

_____

_____

_____

_____

Is there anything I would do differently the following days?

(This could be in regard to your food intake, your discussions about

veganism with others, dealing with difficult scenarios with non-vegans

etc)

_____

_____

_____

_____

_____

_____

_____

MY DAILY VEGAN DIARY

Day 19: _____

How did my day go?

_____
_____
_____
_____
_____
_____
_____
_____
_____
_____
_____
_____
_____
_____
_____
_____
_____
_____
_____
_____
_____
_____
_____
_____
_____
_____
_____

Has my food intake been sufficient in:

Protein ☐　　Calcium ☐　Iron ☐　　Omega 3 ☐　Vitamin C ☐　Fibre ☐

Notes

How has my mood been today?

_____

_____

_____

_____

_____

_____

Is there anything I would do differently the following days?

(This could be in regard to your food intake, your discussions about

veganism with others, dealing with difficult scenarios with non-vegans

etc)

_____

_____

_____

_____

_____

_____

_____

MY DAILY VEGAN DIARY

Day 20.

How did my day go?

_____
_____
_____
_____
_____
_____
_____
_____
_____
_____
_____
_____
_____
_____
_____
_____
_____
_____
_____
_____
_____
_____
_____
_____
_____
_____
_____

Has my food intake been sufficient in:

Protein ☐   Calcium ☐   Iron ☐   Omega 3 ☐   Vitamin C ☐   Fibre ☐

Notes

How has my mood been today?

Is there anything I would do differently the following days?
(This could be in regard to your food intake, your discussions about veganism with others, dealing with difficult scenarios with non-vegans etc)

MY DAILY VEGAN DIARY

Day 21: _____

How did my day go?

_____
_____
_____
_____
_____
_____
_____
_____
_____
_____
_____
_____
_____
_____
_____
_____
_____
_____
_____
_____
_____
_____
_____
_____
_____
_____
_____
_____
_____
_____
_____
_____

Has my food intake been sufficient in:

Protein ☐   Calcium ☐   Iron ☐   Omega 3 ☐   Vitamin C ☐   Fibre ☐

Notes

How has my mood been today?

_____

_____

_____

_____

_____

_____

Is there anything I would do differently the following days?

(This could be in regard to your food intake, your discussions about

veganism with others, dealing with difficult scenarios with non-vegans

etc)

_____

_____

_____

_____

_____

_____

_____

MY DAILY VEGAN DIARY

Day 22: _____

How did my day go?

_____
_____
_____
_____
_____
_____
_____
_____
_____
_____
_____
_____
_____
_____
_____
_____
_____
_____
_____
_____
_____
_____
_____
_____
_____
_____
_____
_____
_____

Has my food intake been sufficient in:

Protein ☐   Calcium ☐   Iron ☐   Omega 3 ☐   Vitamin C ☐   Fibre ☐

Notes

How has my mood been today?

_____

_____

_____

_____

_____

_____

Is there anything I would do differently the following days?

(This could be in regard to your food intake, your discussions about veganism with others, dealing with difficult scenarios with non-vegans etc)

_____

_____

_____

_____

_____

_____

_____

MY DAILY VEGAN DIARY

Day 23.

How did my day go?

_____
_____
_____
_____
_____
_____
_____
_____
_____
_____
_____
_____
_____
_____
_____
_____
_____
_____
_____
_____
_____
_____
_____
_____
_____
_____

Has my food intake been sufficient in:

Protein ☐   Calcium ☐   Iron ☐   Omega 3 ☐   Vitamin C ☐   Fibre ☐

Notes

How has my mood been today?

_____

_____

_____

_____

_____

_____

Is there anything I would do differently the following days?

(This could be in regard to your food intake, your discussions about

veganism with others, dealing with difficult scenarios with non-vegans

etc)

_____

_____

_____

_____

_____

_____

_____

MY DAILY VEGAN DIARY

Day 24: _____

How did my day go?

_____
_____
_____
_____
_____
_____
_____
_____
_____
_____
_____
_____
_____
_____
_____
_____
_____
_____
_____
_____
_____
_____
_____
_____
_____
_____
_____

Has my food intake been sufficient in:

Protein ☐   Calcium ☐   Iron ☐   Omega 3 ☐   Vitamin C ☐   Fibre ☐

Notes

How has my mood been today?

_____

_____

_____

_____

_____

_____

Is there anything I would do differently the following days?

(This could be in regard to your food intake, your discussions about veganism with others, dealing with difficult scenarios with non-vegans etc)

_____

_____

_____

_____

_____

_____

_____

MY DAILY VEGAN DIARY

Day 25.

How did my day go?

_____
_____
_____
_____
_____
_____
_____
_____
_____
_____
_____
_____
_____
_____
_____
_____
_____
_____
_____
_____
_____
_____
_____
_____
_____
_____
_____

Has my food intake been sufficient in:

Protein ☐   Calcium ☐   Iron ☐   Omega 3 ☐   Vitamin C ☐   Fibre ☐

Notes

How has my mood been today?

_____

_____

_____

_____

_____

_____

Is there anything I would do differently the following days?

(This could be in regard to your food intake, your discussions about

veganism with others, dealing with difficult scenarios with non-vegans

etc)

_____

_____

_____

_____

_____

_____

_____

MY DAILY VEGAN DIARY

Day 26: _____

How did my day go?

_____
_____
_____
_____
_____
_____
_____
_____
_____
_____
_____
_____
_____
_____
_____
_____
_____
_____
_____
_____
_____
_____
_____
_____
_____
_____
_____
_____
_____

Has my food intake been sufficient in:

Protein ☐   Calcium ☐   Iron ☐   Omega 3 ☐   Vitamin C ☐   Fibre ☐

Notes

How has my mood been today?

_____

_____

_____

_____

_____

_____

Is there anything I would do differently the following days?

(This could be in regard to your food intake, your discussions about veganism with others, dealing with difficult scenarios with non-vegans etc)

_____

_____

_____

_____

_____

_____

_____

MY DAILY VEGAN DIARY

Day 27. _____

How did my day go?

_____
_____
_____
_____
_____
_____
_____
_____
_____
_____
_____
_____
_____
_____
_____
_____
_____
_____
_____
_____
_____
_____
_____
_____
_____
_____
_____
_____
_____
_____
_____
_____

Has my food intake been sufficient in:

Protein ☐   Calcium ☐   Iron ☐   Omega 3 ☐   Vitamin C ☐   Fibre ☐

Notes

How has my mood been today?

Is there anything I would do differently the following days?

(This could be in regard to your food intake, your discussions about

veganism with others, dealing with difficult scenarios with non-vegans

etc)

MY DAILY VEGAN DIARY

Day 28:

How did my day go?

_____
_____
_____
_____
_____
_____
_____
_____
_____
_____
_____
_____
_____
_____
_____
_____
_____
_____
_____
_____
_____
_____
_____
_____
_____
_____
_____

Has my food intake been sufficient in:

Protein ☐   Calcium ☐   Iron ☐   Omega 3 ☐   Vitamin C ☐   Fibre ☐

Notes

How has my mood been today?

Is there anything I would do differently the following days?
(This could be in regard to your food intake, your discussions about
veganism with others, dealing with difficult scenarios with non-vegans
etc)

MY DAILY VEGAN DIARY

Day 29.

How did my day go?

_____
_____
_____
_____
_____
_____
_____
_____
_____
_____
_____
_____
_____
_____
_____
_____
_____
_____
_____
_____
_____
_____
_____
_____
_____
_____
_____

Has my food intake been sufficient in:

Protein ☐   Calcium ☐   Iron ☐   Omega 3 ☐   Vitamin C ☐   Fibre ☐

Notes

How has my mood been today?

_____
_____
_____
_____
_____
_____

Is there anything I would do differently the following days?

(This could be in regard to your food intake, your discussions about veganism with others, dealing with difficult scenarios with non-vegans etc)

_____
_____
_____
_____
_____
_____
_____

MY DAILY VEGAN DIARY

Day 30.

How did my day go?

_____
_____
_____
_____
_____
_____
_____
_____
_____
_____
_____
_____
_____
_____
_____
_____
_____
_____
_____
_____
_____
_____
_____
_____
_____
_____
_____
_____
_____

Has my food intake been sufficient in:

Protein ☐   Calcium ☐   Iron ☐   Omega 3 ☐   Vitamin C ☐   Fibre ☐

Notes

How has my mood been today?

Is there anything I would do differently the following days?

(This could be in regard to your food intake, your discussions about

veganism with others, dealing with difficult scenarios with non-vegans

etc)

MY DAILY VEGAN DIARY

Day 31: _____

How did my day go?

_____
_____
_____
_____
_____
_____
_____
_____
_____
_____
_____
_____
_____
_____
_____
_____
_____
_____
_____
_____
_____
_____
_____
_____
_____
_____
_____
_____

Has my food intake been sufficient in:

Protein ☐   Calcium ☐   Iron ☐   Omega 3 ☐   Vitamin C ☐   Fibre ☐

Notes

How has my mood been today?

_____

_____

_____

_____

_____

_____

Is there anything I would do differently the following days?

(This could be in regard to your food intake, your discussions about veganism with others, dealing with difficult scenarios with non-vegans etc)

_____

_____

_____

_____

_____

_____

_____

MY DAILY VEGAN DIARY

Day 32

How did my day go?

_____
_____
_____
_____
_____
_____
_____
_____
_____
_____
_____
_____
_____
_____
_____
_____
_____
_____
_____
_____
_____
_____
_____
_____
_____
_____

Has my food intake been sufficient in:

Protein ☐   Calcium ☐   Iron ☐   Omega 3 ☐   Vitamin C ☐   Fibre ☐

Notes

How has my mood been today?

Is there anything I would do differently the following days?
(This could be in regard to your food intake, your discussions about veganism with others, dealing with difficult scenarios with non-vegans etc)

MY DAILY VEGAN DIARY

Day 33: _____

How did my day go?

_____
_____
_____
_____
_____
_____
_____
_____
_____
_____
_____
_____
_____
_____
_____
_____
_____
_____
_____
_____
_____
_____
_____
_____
_____
_____
_____
_____

Has my food intake been sufficient in:

Protein ☐   Calcium ☐   Iron ☐   Omega 3 ☐   Vitamin C ☐   Fibre ☐

Notes

How has my mood been today?

_____

_____

_____

_____

_____

_____

Is there anything I would do differently the following days?

(This could be in regard to your food intake, your discussions about

veganism with others, dealing with difficult scenarios with non-vegans

etc)

_____

_____

_____

_____

_____

_____

_____

MY DAILY VEGAN DIARY

Day 34.

How did my day go?

_____
_____
_____
_____
_____
_____
_____
_____
_____
_____
_____
_____
_____
_____
_____
_____
_____
_____
_____
_____
_____
_____
_____
_____
_____
_____

Has my food intake been sufficient in:

Protein ☐   Calcium ☐   Iron ☐   Omega 3 ☐   Vitamin C ☐   Fibre ☐

Notes

How has my mood been today?

Is there anything I would do differently the following days?
(This could be in regard to your food intake, your discussions about veganism with others, dealing with difficult scenarios with non-vegans etc)

MY DAILY VEGAN DIARY

Day 35: _____

How did my day go?

_____
_____
_____
_____
_____
_____
_____
_____
_____
_____
_____
_____
_____
_____
_____
_____
_____
_____
_____
_____
_____
_____
_____
_____
_____
_____
_____
_____

Has my food intake been sufficient in:

Protein ☐   Calcium ☐   Iron ☐   Omega 3 ☐   Vitamin C ☐   Fibre ☐

Notes

How has my mood been today?

_____

_____

_____

_____

_____

_____

Is there anything I would do differently the following days?

(This could be in regard to your food intake, your discussions about veganism with others, dealing with difficult scenarios with non-vegans etc)

_____

_____

_____

_____

_____

_____

_____

MY DAILY VEGAN DIARY

Day 36.

How did my day go?

_____
_____
_____
_____
_____
_____
_____
_____
_____
_____
_____
_____
_____
_____
_____
_____
_____
_____
_____
_____
_____
_____
_____
_____
_____
_____
_____
_____
_____

Has my food intake been sufficient in:

Protein ☐   Calcium ☐   Iron ☐   Omega 3 ☐   Vitamin C ☐   Fibre ☐

Notes

How has my mood been today?

_____
_____
_____
_____
_____
_____

Is there anything I would do differently the following days?
(This could be in regard to your food intake, your discussions about veganism with others, dealing with difficult scenarios with non-vegans etc)

_____
_____
_____
_____
_____
_____

MY DAILY VEGAN DIARY

Day 37: _____

How did my day go?

_____
_____
_____
_____
_____
_____
_____
_____
_____
_____
_____
_____
_____
_____
_____
_____
_____
_____
_____
_____
_____
_____
_____
_____
_____
_____
_____
_____
_____

Has my food intake been sufficient in:

Protein ☐   Calcium ☐   Iron ☐   Omega 3 ☐   Vitamin C ☐   Fibre ☐

Notes

How has my mood been today?

_____
_____
_____
_____
_____
_____

Is there anything I would do differently the following days?

(This could be in regard to your food intake, your discussions about

veganism with others, dealing with difficult scenarios with non-vegans

etc)

_____
_____
_____
_____
_____
_____
_____

MY DAILY VEGAN DIARY

Day 38.

How did my day go?

_____
_____
_____
_____
_____
_____
_____
_____
_____
_____
_____
_____
_____
_____
_____
_____
_____
_____
_____
_____
_____
_____
_____
_____
_____
_____
_____

Has my food intake been sufficient in:

Protein ☐   Calcium ☐   Iron ☐   Omega 3 ☐   Vitamin C ☐   Fibre ☐

Notes

How has my mood been today?

_____

_____

_____

_____

_____

_____

Is there anything I would do differently the following days?

(This could be in regard to your food intake, your discussions about

veganism with others, dealing with difficult scenarios with non-vegans

etc)

_____

_____

_____

_____

_____

_____

_____

MY DAILY VEGAN DIARY

Day 39. _____

How did my day go?

_____
_____
_____
_____
_____
_____
_____
_____
_____
_____
_____
_____
_____
_____
_____
_____
_____
_____
_____
_____
_____
_____
_____
_____
_____
_____
_____
_____

Has my food intake been sufficient in:

Protein ☐   Calcium ☐   Iron ☐   Omega 3 ☐   Vitamin C ☐   Fibre ☐

Notes

How has my mood been today?

_____

_____

_____

_____

_____

_____

Is there anything I would do differently the following days?
(This could be in regard to your food intake, your discussions about veganism with others, dealing with difficult scenarios with non-vegans etc)

_____

_____

_____

_____

_____

_____

_____

MY DAILY VEGAN DIARY

Day 40: _____

How did my day go?

_____
_____
_____
_____
_____
_____
_____
_____
_____
_____
_____
_____
_____
_____
_____
_____
_____
_____
_____
_____
_____
_____
_____
_____
_____
_____
_____
_____
_____
_____

Has my food intake been sufficient in:

Protein ☐   Calcium ☐   Iron ☐   Omega 3 ☐   Vitamin C ☐   Fibre ☐

Notes

How has my mood been today?

_____
_____
_____
_____
_____
_____

Is there anything I would do differently the following days?

(This could be in regard to your food intake, your discussions about veganism with others, dealing with difficult scenarios with non-vegans etc)

_____
_____
_____
_____
_____
_____

MY DAILY VEGAN DIARY

Day 41: _____

How did my day go?

_____
_____
_____
_____
_____
_____
_____
_____
_____
_____
_____
_____
_____
_____
_____
_____
_____
_____
_____
_____
_____
_____
_____
_____
_____
_____
_____
_____

Has my food intake been sufficient in:

Protein ☐   Calcium ☐   Iron ☐   Omega 3 ☐   Vitamin C ☐   Fibre ☐

Notes

How has my mood been today?

_____
_____
_____
_____
_____
_____

Is there anything I would do differently the following days?
(This could be in regard to your food intake, your discussions about veganism with others, dealing with difficult scenarios with non-vegans etc)

_____
_____
_____
_____
_____
_____

MY DAILY VEGAN DIARY

Day 42.

How did my day go?

_____
_____
_____
_____
_____
_____
_____
_____
_____
_____
_____
_____
_____
_____
_____
_____
_____
_____
_____
_____
_____
_____
_____
_____
_____
_____
_____

Has my food intake been sufficient in:

Protein ☐   Calcium ☐   Iron ☐   Omega 3 ☐   Vitamin C ☐   Fibre ☐

Notes

How has my mood been today?

_____
_____
_____
_____
_____
_____

Is there anything I would do differently the following days?
(This could be in regard to your food intake, your discussions about veganism with others, dealing with difficult scenarios with non-vegans etc)

_____
_____
_____
_____
_____
_____

MY DAILY VEGAN DIARY

Day 43:_____

How did my day go?

_____
_____
_____
_____
_____
_____
_____
_____
_____
_____
_____
_____
_____
_____
_____
_____
_____
_____
_____
_____
_____
_____
_____
_____
_____
_____
_____
_____

Has my food intake been sufficient in:

Protein ☐   Calcium ☐   Iron ☐   Omega 3 ☐   Vitamin C ☐   Fibre ☐

Notes

How has my mood been today?

_____

_____

_____

_____

_____

_____

Is there anything I would do differently the following days?

(This could be in regard to your food intake, your discussions about

veganism with others, dealing with difficult scenarios with non-vegans

etc)

_____

_____

_____

_____

_____

_____

MY DAILY VEGAN DIARY

Day 44

How did my day go?

_____
_____
_____
_____
_____
_____
_____
_____
_____
_____
_____
_____
_____
_____
_____
_____
_____
_____
_____
_____
_____
_____
_____
_____
_____
_____

Has my food intake been sufficient in:

Protein ☐   Calcium ☐   Iron ☐   Omega 3 ☐   Vitamin C ☐   Fibre ☐

Notes

How has my mood been today?

Is there anything I would do differently the following days?
(This could be in regard to your food intake, your discussions about veganism with others, dealing with difficult scenarios with non-vegans etc)

MY DAILY VEGAN DIARY

Day 45:

How did my day go?

_____
_____
_____
_____
_____
_____
_____
_____
_____
_____
_____
_____
_____
_____
_____
_____
_____
_____
_____
_____
_____
_____
_____
_____
_____
_____
_____
_____
_____

Has my food intake been sufficient in:

Protein ☐   Calcium ☐   Iron ☐   Omega 3 ☐   Vitamin C ☐   Fibre ☐

Notes

How has my mood been today?

_____

_____

_____

_____

_____

_____

Is there anything I would do differently the following days?

(This could be in regard to your food intake, your discussions about

veganism with others, dealing with difficult scenarios with non-vegans

etc)

_____

_____

_____

_____

_____

_____

_____

MY DAILY VEGAN DIARY

Day 46: _____

How did my day go?

_____
_____
_____
_____
_____
_____
_____
_____
_____
_____
_____
_____
_____
_____
_____
_____
_____
_____
_____
_____
_____
_____
_____
_____
_____
_____
_____
_____

Has my food intake been sufficient in:

Protein ☐   Calcium ☐   Iron ☐   Omega 3 ☐   Vitamin C ☐   Fibre ☐

Notes

How has my mood been today?

Is there anything I would do differently the following days?
(This could be in regard to your food intake, your discussions about veganism with others, dealing with difficult scenarios with non-vegans etc)

MY DAILY VEGAN DIARY

Day 47: _____

How did my day go?

_____
_____
_____
_____
_____
_____
_____
_____
_____
_____
_____
_____
_____
_____
_____
_____
_____
_____
_____
_____
_____
_____
_____
_____
_____
_____
_____

Has my food intake been sufficient in:

Protein ☐   Calcium ☐   Iron ☐   Omega 3 ☐   Vitamin C ☐   Fibre ☐

Notes

How has my mood been today?

_____

_____

_____

_____

_____

_____

Is there anything I would do differently the following days?

(This could be in regard to your food intake, your discussions about veganism with others, dealing with difficult scenarios with non-vegans etc)

_____

_____

_____

_____

_____

_____

_____

MY DAILY VEGAN DIARY

Day 48: _____

How did my day go?

_____
_____
_____
_____
_____
_____
_____
_____
_____
_____
_____
_____
_____
_____
_____
_____
_____
_____
_____
_____
_____
_____
_____
_____
_____
_____

Has my food intake been sufficient in:

Protein ☐   Calcium ☐   Iron ☐   Omega 3 ☐   Vitamin C ☐   Fibre ☐

Notes

How has my mood been today?

_____
_____
_____
_____
_____
_____

Is there anything I would do differently the following days?
(This could be in regard to your food intake, your discussions about veganism with others, dealing with difficult scenarios with non-vegans etc)

_____
_____
_____
_____
_____
_____
_____

MY DAILY VEGAN DIARY

Day 49.

How did my day go?

_____
_____
_____
_____
_____
_____
_____
_____
_____
_____
_____
_____
_____
_____
_____
_____
_____
_____
_____
_____
_____
_____
_____
_____
_____
_____
_____

Has my food intake been sufficient in:

Protein ☐   Calcium ☐   Iron ☐   Omega 3 ☐   Vitamin C ☐   Fibre ☐

Notes

How has my mood been today?

_____
_____
_____
_____
_____
_____

Is there anything I would do differently the following days?
(This could be in regard to your food intake, your discussions about veganism with others, dealing with difficult scenarios with non-vegans etc)

_____
_____
_____
_____
_____
_____
_____

MY DAILY VEGAN DIARY

Day 50:

How did my day go?

_____
_____
_____
_____
_____
_____
_____
_____
_____
_____
_____
_____
_____
_____
_____
_____
_____
_____
_____
_____
_____
_____
_____
_____
_____
_____
_____
_____

Has my food intake been sufficient in:

Protein ☐   Calcium ☐   Iron ☐   Omega 3 ☐   Vitamin C ☐   Fibre ☐

Notes

How has my mood been today?

_____

_____

_____

_____

_____

Is there anything I would do differently the following days?
(This could be in regard to your food intake, your discussions about veganism with others, dealing with difficult scenarios with non-vegans etc)

_____

_____

_____

_____

_____

_____

MY DAILY VEGAN DIARY

Day 51. _____

How did my day go?

_____
_____
_____
_____
_____
_____
_____
_____
_____
_____
_____
_____
_____
_____
_____
_____
_____
_____
_____
_____
_____
_____
_____
_____
_____
_____
_____
_____
_____
_____

Has my food intake been sufficient in:

Protein ☐   Calcium ☐   Iron ☐   Omega 3 ☐   Vitamin C ☐   Fibre ☐

Notes

How has my mood been today?

_____

_____

_____

_____

_____

_____

Is there anything I would do differently the following days?

(This could be in regard to your food intake, your discussions about veganism with others, dealing with difficult scenarios with non-vegans etc)

_____

_____

_____

_____

_____

_____

_____

MY DAILY VEGAN DIARY

Day 52:

How did my day go?

_____
_____
_____
_____
_____
_____
_____
_____
_____
_____
_____
_____
_____
_____
_____
_____
_____
_____
_____
_____
_____
_____
_____
_____
_____
_____
_____
_____

Has my food intake been sufficient in:

Protein ☐   Calcium ☐   Iron ☐   Omega 3 ☐   Vitamin C ☐   Fibre ☐

Notes

How has my mood been today?

_____
_____
_____
_____
_____
_____

Is there anything I would do differently the following days?
(This could be in regard to your food intake, your discussions about veganism with others, dealing with difficult scenarios with non-vegans etc)

_____
_____
_____
_____
_____
_____
_____

MY DAILY VEGAN DIARY

Day 53

How did my day go?

_____
_____
_____
_____
_____
_____
_____
_____
_____
_____
_____
_____
_____
_____
_____
_____
_____
_____
_____
_____
_____
_____
_____
_____
_____
_____
_____

Has my food intake been sufficient in:

Protein ☐   Calcium ☐   Iron ☐   Omega 3 ☐   Vitamin C ☐   Fibre ☐

Notes

How has my mood been today?

_____

_____

_____

_____

_____

_____

Is there anything I would do differently the following days?
(This could be in regard to your food intake, your discussions about veganism with others, dealing with difficult scenarios with non-vegans etc)

_____

_____

_____

_____

_____

_____

_____

MY DAILY VEGAN DIARY

Day 54: _____

How did my day go?

_____
_____
_____
_____
_____
_____
_____
_____
_____
_____
_____
_____
_____
_____
_____
_____
_____
_____
_____
_____
_____
_____
_____
_____

Has my food intake been sufficient in:

Protein ☐   Calcium ☐   Iron ☐   Omega 3 ☐   Vitamin C ☐   Fibre ☐

Notes

How has my mood been today?

_____
_____
_____
_____
_____
_____

Is there anything I would do differently the following days?
(This could be in regard to your food intake, your discussions about veganism with others, dealing with difficult scenarios with non-vegans etc)

_____
_____
_____
_____
_____
_____
_____

MY DAILY VEGAN DIARY

Day 55: _____

How did my day go?

_____
_____
_____
_____
_____
_____
_____
_____
_____
_____
_____
_____
_____
_____
_____
_____
_____
_____
_____
_____
_____
_____
_____
_____
_____
_____
_____
_____

Has my food intake been sufficient in:

Protein ☐   Calcium ☐   Iron ☐   Omega 3 ☐   Vitamin C ☐   Fibre ☐

Notes

How has my mood been today?

_____
_____
_____
_____
_____
_____

Is there anything I would do differently the following days?

(This could be in regard to your food intake, your discussions about veganism with others, dealing with difficult scenarios with non-vegans etc)

_____
_____
_____
_____
_____
_____
_____

MY DAILY VEGAN DIARY

Day 56:

How did my day go?

_____
_____
_____
_____
_____
_____
_____
_____
_____
_____
_____
_____
_____
_____
_____
_____
_____
_____
_____
_____
_____
_____
_____
_____
_____
_____
_____

Has my food intake been sufficient in:

Protein ☐   Calcium ☐   Iron ☐   Omega 3 ☐   Vitamin C ☐   Fibre ☐

Notes

How has my mood been today?

_____

_____

_____

_____

_____

_____

Is there anything I would do differently the following days?

(This could be in regard to your food intake, your discussions about veganism with others, dealing with difficult scenarios with non-vegans etc)

_____

_____

_____

_____

_____

_____

_____

MY DAILY VEGAN DIARY

Day 57:

How did my day go?

_____
_____
_____
_____
_____
_____
_____
_____
_____
_____
_____
_____
_____
_____
_____
_____
_____
_____
_____
_____
_____
_____
_____
_____
_____
_____
_____
_____
_____

Has my food intake been sufficient in:

Protein ☐   Calcium ☐   Iron ☐   Omega 3 ☐   Vitamin C ☐   Fibre ☐

Notes

How has my mood been today?

_____

_____

_____

_____

_____

_____

Is there anything I would do differently the following days?

(This could be in regard to your food intake, your discussions about

veganism with others, dealing with difficult scenarios with non-vegans

etc)

_____

_____

_____

_____

_____

_____

_____

MY DAILY VEGAN DIARY

Day 58

How did my day go?

_____
_____
_____
_____
_____
_____
_____
_____
_____
_____
_____
_____
_____
_____
_____
_____
_____
_____
_____
_____
_____
_____
_____
_____
_____
_____
_____
_____

Has my food intake been sufficient in:

Protein ☐   Calcium ☐   Iron ☐   Omega 3 ☐   Vitamin C ☐   Fibre ☐

Notes

How has my mood been today?

_____
_____
_____
_____
_____
_____

Is there anything I would do differently the following days?
(This could be in regard to your food intake, your discussions about
veganism with others, dealing with difficult scenarios with non-vegans
etc)

_____
_____
_____
_____
_____
_____
_____

MY DAILY VEGAN DIARY

Day 59:

How did my day go?

_____
_____
_____
_____
_____
_____
_____
_____
_____
_____
_____
_____
_____
_____
_____
_____
_____
_____
_____
_____
_____
_____
_____
_____
_____
_____
_____
_____

Has my food intake been sufficient in:

Protein ☐   Calcium ☐   Iron ☐   Omega 3 ☐   Vitamin C ☐   Fibre ☐

Notes

How has my mood been today?

_____

_____

_____

_____

_____

_____

Is there anything I would do differently the following days?

(This could be in regard to your food intake, your discussions about

veganism with others, dealing with difficult scenarios with non-vegans

etc)

_____

_____

_____

_____

_____

_____

_____

MY DAILY VEGAN DIARY

Day 60: _____

How did my day go?

_____
_____
_____
_____
_____
_____
_____
_____
_____
_____
_____
_____
_____
_____
_____
_____
_____
_____
_____
_____
_____
_____
_____
_____
_____
_____
_____
_____

Has my food intake been sufficient in:

Protein ☐   Calcium ☐   Iron ☐   Omega 3 ☐   Vitamin C ☐   Fibre ☐

Notes

How has my mood been today?

_____

_____

_____

_____

_____

Is there anything I would do differently the following days?

(This could be in regard to your food intake, your discussions about

veganism with others, dealing with difficult scenarios with non-vegans

etc)

_____

_____

_____

_____

_____

_____

MY DAILY VEGAN DIARY

Day 61: _____

How did my day go?

_____
_____
_____
_____
_____
_____
_____
_____
_____
_____
_____
_____
_____
_____
_____
_____
_____
_____
_____
_____
_____
_____
_____
_____
_____
_____
_____
_____
_____
_____

Has my food intake been sufficient in:

Protein ☐   Calcium ☐   Iron ☐   Omega 3 ☐   Vitamin C ☐   Fibre ☐

Notes

How has my mood been today?

_____

_____

_____

_____

_____

_____

Is there anything I would do differently the following days?
(This could be in regard to your food intake, your discussions about veganism with others, dealing with difficult scenarios with non-vegans etc)

_____

_____

_____

_____

_____

_____

_____

MY DAILY VEGAN DIARY

Day 62: _____

How did my day go?

_____
_____
_____
_____
_____
_____
_____
_____
_____
_____
_____
_____
_____
_____
_____
_____
_____
_____
_____
_____
_____
_____
_____
_____
_____
_____
_____

Has my food intake been sufficient in:

Protein ☐   Calcium ☐   Iron ☐   Omega 3 ☐   Vitamin C ☐   Fibre ☐

Notes

How has my mood been today?

_____

_____

_____

_____

_____

_____

Is there anything I would do differently the following days?

(This could be in regard to your food intake, your discussions about

veganism with others, dealing with difficult scenarios with non-vegans

etc)

_____

_____

_____

_____

_____

_____

_____

MY DAILY VEGAN DIARY

Day 63

How did my day go?

_____
_____
_____
_____
_____
_____
_____
_____
_____
_____
_____
_____
_____
_____
_____
_____
_____
_____
_____
_____
_____
_____
_____
_____
_____
_____
_____
_____

Has my food intake been sufficient in:

Protein ☐   Calcium ☐   Iron ☐   Omega 3 ☐   Vitamin C ☐   Fibre ☐

Notes

How has my mood been today?

_____

_____

_____

_____

_____

_____

Is there anything I would do differently the following days?

(This could be in regard to your food intake, your discussions about veganism with others, dealing with difficult scenarios with non-vegans etc)

_____

_____

_____

_____

_____

_____

MY DAILY VEGAN DIARY

Day 64

How did my day go?

_____
_____
_____
_____
_____
_____
_____
_____
_____
_____
_____
_____
_____
_____
_____
_____
_____
_____
_____
_____
_____
_____
_____
_____
_____
_____
_____
_____
_____

Has my food intake been sufficient in:

Protein ☐   Calcium ☐   Iron ☐   Omega 3 ☐   Vitamin C ☐   Fibre ☐

Notes

How has my mood been today?

_____
_____
_____
_____
_____
_____

Is there anything I would do differently the following days?

(This could be in regard to your food intake, your discussions about

veganism with others, dealing with difficult scenarios with non-vegans

etc)

_____
_____
_____
_____
_____
_____
_____

MY DAILY VEGAN DIARY

Day 65.

How did my day go?

_____
_____
_____
_____
_____
_____
_____
_____
_____
_____
_____
_____
_____
_____
_____
_____
_____
_____
_____
_____
_____
_____
_____
_____
_____
_____
_____
_____

Has my food intake been sufficient in:

Protein ☐   Calcium ☐   Iron ☐   Omega 3 ☐   Vitamin C ☐   Fibre ☐

Notes

How has my mood been today?

_____

_____

_____

_____

_____

Is there anything I would do differently the following days?

(This could be in regard to your food intake, your discussions about

veganism with others, dealing with difficult scenarios with non-vegans

etc)

_____

_____

_____

_____

_____

_____

_____

MY DAILY VEGAN DIARY

*Day 66:*_____

How did my day go?

_____
_____
_____
_____
_____
_____
_____
_____
_____
_____
_____
_____
_____
_____
_____
_____
_____
_____
_____
_____
_____
_____
_____
_____
_____
_____
_____
_____
_____
_____
_____

Has my food intake been sufficient in:

Protein ☐   Calcium ☐   Iron ☐   Omega 3 ☐   Vitamin C ☐   Fibre ☐

Notes

How has my mood been today?

_____

_____

_____

_____

_____

_____

Is there anything I would do differently the following days?

(This could be in regard to your food intake, your discussions about veganism with others, dealing with difficult scenarios with non-vegans etc)

_____

_____

_____

_____

_____

_____

_____

MY DAILY VEGAN DIARY

Day 67.

How did my day go?

_____
_____
_____
_____
_____
_____
_____
_____
_____
_____
_____
_____
_____
_____
_____
_____
_____
_____
_____
_____
_____
_____
_____
_____
_____
_____
_____

Has my food intake been sufficient in:

Protein ☐   Calcium ☐   Iron ☐   Omega 3 ☐   Vitamin C ☐   Fibre ☐

Notes

How has my mood been today?

_____

_____

_____

_____

_____

_____

Is there anything I would do differently the following days?

(This could be in regard to your food intake, your discussions about veganism with others, dealing with difficult scenarios with non-vegans etc)

_____

_____

_____

_____

_____

_____

_____

MY DAILY VEGAN DIARY

Day 68: _____

How did my day go?

_____
_____
_____
_____
_____
_____
_____
_____
_____
_____
_____
_____
_____
_____
_____
_____
_____
_____
_____
_____
_____
_____
_____
_____
_____
_____
_____
_____

Has my food intake been sufficient in:

Protein ☐   Calcium ☐   Iron ☐   Omega 3 ☐   Vitamin C ☐   Fibre ☐

Notes

How has my mood been today?

_____
_____
_____
_____
_____
_____

Is there anything I would do differently the following days?
(This could be in regard to your food intake, your discussions about veganism with others, dealing with difficult scenarios with non-vegans etc)

_____
_____
_____
_____
_____
_____
_____

MY DAILY VEGAN DIARY

Day 69: _____

How did my day go?

_____
_____
_____
_____
_____
_____
_____
_____
_____
_____
_____
_____
_____
_____
_____
_____
_____
_____
_____
_____
_____
_____
_____
_____
_____
_____
_____

Has my food intake been sufficient in:

Protein ☐   Calcium ☐   Iron ☐   Omega 3 ☐   Vitamin C ☐   Fibre ☐

Notes

How has my mood been today?

_____

_____

_____

_____

_____

_____

Is there anything I would do differently the following days?

(This could be in regard to your food intake, your discussions about

veganism with others, dealing with difficult scenarios with non-vegans

etc)

_____

_____

_____

_____

_____

_____

_____

MY DAILY VEGAN DIARY

Day 70:

How did my day go?

_____
_____
_____
_____
_____
_____
_____
_____
_____
_____
_____
_____
_____
_____
_____
_____
_____
_____
_____
_____
_____
_____
_____
_____
_____
_____

Has my food intake been sufficient in:

Protein ☐   Calcium ☐   Iron ☐   Omega 3 ☐   Vitamin C ☐   Fibre ☐

Notes

How has my mood been today?

_____
_____
_____
_____
_____
_____

Is there anything I would do differently the following days?
(This could be in regard to your food intake, your discussions about veganism with others, dealing with difficult scenarios with non-vegans etc)

_____
_____
_____
_____
_____
_____
_____

MY DAILY VEGAN DIARY

Day 71:

How did my day go?

_____
_____
_____
_____
_____
_____
_____
_____
_____
_____
_____
_____
_____
_____
_____
_____
_____
_____
_____
_____
_____
_____
_____
_____
_____
_____

Has my food intake been sufficient in:

Protein ☐   Calcium ☐   Iron ☐   Omega 3 ☐   Vitamin C ☐   Fibre ☐

Notes

How has my mood been today?

_____
_____
_____
_____
_____
_____

Is there anything I would do differently the following days?
(This could be in regard to your food intake, your discussions about veganism with others, dealing with difficult scenarios with non-vegans etc)

_____
_____
_____
_____
_____
_____
_____

MY DAILY VEGAN DIARY

Day 72: _____

How did my day go?

_____
_____
_____
_____
_____
_____
_____
_____
_____
_____
_____
_____
_____
_____
_____
_____
_____
_____
_____
_____
_____
_____
_____
_____
_____
_____
_____
_____
_____
_____

Has my food intake been sufficient in:

Protein ☐   Calcium ☐   Iron ☐   Omega 3 ☐   Vitamin C ☐   Fibre ☐

Notes

How has my mood been today?

_____

_____

_____

_____

_____

_____

Is there anything I would do differently the following days?
(This could be in regard to your food intake, your discussions about
veganism with others, dealing with difficult scenarios with non-vegans
etc)

_____

_____

_____

_____

_____

_____

_____

MY DAILY VEGAN DIARY

Day 73 _____

How did my day go?

_____
_____
_____
_____
_____
_____
_____
_____
_____
_____
_____
_____
_____
_____
_____
_____
_____
_____
_____
_____
_____
_____
_____
_____
_____
_____
_____
_____
_____
_____
_____

Has my food intake been sufficient in:

Protein ☐   Calcium ☐   Iron ☐   Omega 3 ☐   Vitamin C ☐   Fibre ☐

Notes

How has my mood been today?

_____
_____
_____
_____
_____
_____

Is there anything I would do differently the following days?
(This could be in regard to your food intake, your discussions about veganism with others, dealing with difficult scenarios with non-vegans etc)

_____
_____
_____
_____
_____
_____
_____

MY DAILY VEGAN DIARY

Day 74.

How did my day go?

_____
_____
_____
_____
_____
_____
_____
_____
_____
_____
_____
_____
_____
_____
_____
_____
_____
_____
_____
_____
_____
_____
_____
_____
_____

Has my food intake been sufficient in:

Protein ☐   Calcium ☐   Iron ☐   Omega 3 ☐   Vitamin C ☐   Fibre ☐

Notes

How has my mood been today?

_____

_____

_____

_____

_____

_____

Is there anything I would do differently the following days?
(This could be in regard to your food intake, your discussions about veganism with others, dealing with difficult scenarios with non-vegans etc)

_____

_____

_____

_____

_____

_____

_____

MY DAILY VEGAN DIARY

Day 75: _____

How did my day go?

_____
_____
_____
_____
_____
_____
_____
_____
_____
_____
_____
_____
_____
_____
_____
_____
_____
_____
_____
_____
_____
_____
_____
_____
_____
_____
_____
_____

Has my food intake been sufficient in:

Protein ☐   Calcium ☐   Iron ☐   Omega 3 ☐   Vitamin C ☐   Fibre ☐

Notes

How has my mood been today?

Is there anything I would do differently the following days?
(This could be in regard to your food intake, your discussions about veganism with others, dealing with difficult scenarios with non-vegans etc)

MY DAILY VEGAN DIARY

Day 76:

How did my day go?

_____
_____
_____
_____
_____
_____
_____
_____
_____
_____
_____
_____
_____
_____
_____
_____
_____
_____
_____
_____
_____
_____
_____
_____
_____
_____
_____

Has my food intake been sufficient in:

Protein ☐   Calcium ☐   Iron ☐   Omega 3 ☐   Vitamin C ☐   Fibre ☐

Notes

How has my mood been today?

Is there anything I would do differently the following days?
(This could be in regard to your food intake, your discussions about veganism with others, dealing with difficult scenarios with non-vegans etc)

MY DAILY VEGAN DIARY

Day 77: _____

How did my day go?

_____
_____
_____
_____
_____
_____
_____
_____
_____
_____
_____
_____
_____
_____
_____
_____
_____
_____
_____
_____
_____
_____
_____
_____
_____
_____
_____

Has my food intake been sufficient in:

Protein ☐   Calcium ☐   Iron ☐   Omega 3 ☐   Vitamin C ☐   Fibre ☐

Notes

How has my mood been today?

_____

_____

_____

_____

_____

_____

Is there anything I would do differently the following days?

(This could be in regard to your food intake, your discussions about veganism with others, dealing with difficult scenarios with non-vegans etc)

_____

_____

_____

_____

_____

_____

_____

MY DAILY VEGAN DIARY

Day 78: _____

How did my day go?

_____
_____
_____
_____
_____
_____
_____
_____
_____
_____
_____
_____
_____
_____
_____
_____
_____
_____
_____
_____
_____
_____
_____
_____
_____
_____
_____
_____

Has my food intake been sufficient in:

Protein ☐   Calcium ☐   Iron ☐   Omega 3 ☐   Vitamin C ☐   Fibre ☐

Notes

How has my mood been today?

_____
_____
_____
_____
_____
_____

Is there anything I would do differently the following days?
(This could be in regard to your food intake, your discussions about veganism with others, dealing with difficult scenarios with non-vegans etc)

_____
_____
_____
_____
_____
_____
_____

MY DAILY VEGAN DIARY

Day 79: _____

How did my day go?

_____
_____
_____
_____
_____
_____
_____
_____
_____
_____
_____
_____
_____
_____
_____
_____
_____
_____
_____
_____
_____
_____
_____
_____
_____
_____
_____
_____

Has my food intake been sufficient in:

Protein ☐   Calcium ☐   Iron ☐   Omega 3 ☐   Vitamin C ☐   Fibre ☐

Notes

How has my mood been today?

_____
_____
_____
_____
_____
_____

Is there anything I would do differently the following days?
(This could be in regard to your food intake, your discussions about veganism with others, dealing with difficult scenarios with non-vegans etc)

_____
_____
_____
_____
_____
_____
_____

MY DAILY VEGAN DIARY

Day 80.

How did my day go?

_____
_____
_____
_____
_____
_____
_____
_____
_____
_____
_____
_____
_____
_____
_____
_____
_____
_____
_____
_____
_____
_____
_____
_____
_____
_____
_____

Has my food intake been sufficient in:

Protein ☐   Calcium ☐   Iron ☐   Omega 3 ☐   Vitamin C ☐   Fibre ☐

Notes

How has my mood been today?

_____
_____
_____
_____
_____
_____

Is there anything I would do differently the following days?

(This could be in regard to your food intake, your discussions about veganism with others, dealing with difficult scenarios with non-vegans etc)

_____
_____
_____
_____
_____
_____
_____

MY DAILY VEGAN DIARY

Day 81: _____

How did my day go?

_____
_____
_____
_____
_____
_____
_____
_____
_____
_____
_____
_____
_____
_____
_____
_____
_____
_____
_____
_____
_____
_____
_____
_____
_____
_____
_____
_____
_____

Has my food intake been sufficient in:

Protein ☐   Calcium ☐   Iron ☐   Omega 3 ☐   Vitamin C ☐   Fibre ☐

Notes

How has my mood been today?

_____

_____

_____

_____

_____

_____

Is there anything I would do differently the following days?

(This could be in regard to your food intake, your discussions about veganism with others, dealing with difficult scenarios with non-vegans etc)

_____

_____

_____

_____

_____

_____

MY DAILY VEGAN DIARY

Day 82

How did my day go?

_____
_____
_____
_____
_____
_____
_____
_____
_____
_____
_____
_____
_____
_____
_____
_____
_____
_____
_____
_____
_____
_____
_____
_____
_____
_____

Has my food intake been sufficient in:

Protein ☐   Calcium ☐   Iron ☐   Omega 3 ☐   Vitamin C ☐   Fibre ☐

Notes

How has my mood been today?

Is there anything I would do differently the following days?
(This could be in regard to your food intake, your discussions about veganism with others, dealing with difficult scenarios with non-vegans etc)

MY DAILY VEGAN DIARY

Day 83:

How did my day go?

_____
_____
_____
_____
_____
_____
_____
_____
_____
_____
_____
_____
_____
_____
_____
_____
_____
_____
_____
_____
_____
_____
_____
_____
_____
_____
_____
_____
_____

Has my food intake been sufficient in:

Protein ☐   Calcium ☐   Iron ☐   Omega 3 ☐   Vitamin C ☐   Fibre ☐

Notes

How has my mood been today?

_____

_____

_____

_____

_____

_____

Is there anything I would do differently the following days?

(This could be in regard to your food intake, your discussions about veganism with others, dealing with difficult scenarios with non-vegans etc)

_____

_____

_____

_____

_____

_____

_____

MY DAILY VEGAN DIARY

Day 84: _____

How did my day go?

_____
_____
_____
_____
_____
_____
_____
_____
_____
_____
_____
_____
_____
_____
_____
_____
_____
_____
_____
_____
_____
_____
_____
_____
_____
_____
_____

Has my food intake been sufficient in:

Protein ☐   Calcium ☐   Iron ☐   Omega 3 ☐   Vitamin C ☐   Fibre ☐

Notes

How has my mood been today?

_____
_____
_____
_____
_____
_____

Is there anything I would do differently the following days?

(This could be in regard to your food intake, your discussions about

veganism with others, dealing with difficult scenarios with non-vegans

etc)

_____
_____
_____
_____
_____
_____
_____

MY DAILY VEGAN DIARY

Day 85: _____

How did my day go?

_____
_____
_____
_____
_____
_____
_____
_____
_____
_____
_____
_____
_____
_____
_____
_____
_____
_____
_____
_____
_____
_____
_____
_____
_____
_____
_____
_____
_____
_____
_____

Has my food intake been sufficient in:

Protein ☐   Calcium ☐   Iron ☐   Omega 3 ☐   Vitamin C ☐   Fibre ☐

Notes

How has my mood been today?

Is there anything I would do differently the following days?
(This could be in regard to your food intake, your discussions about veganism with others, dealing with difficult scenarios with non-vegans etc)

MY DAILY VEGAN DIARY

Day 86: _____

How did my day go?

_____
_____
_____
_____
_____
_____
_____
_____
_____
_____
_____
_____
_____
_____
_____
_____
_____
_____
_____
_____
_____
_____
_____
_____
_____
_____
_____

Has my food intake been sufficient in:

Protein ☐   Calcium ☐   Iron ☐   Omega 3 ☐   Vitamin C ☐   Fibre ☐

Notes

How has my mood been today?

_____
_____
_____
_____
_____
_____

Is there anything I would do differently the following days?
(This could be in regard to your food intake, your discussions about veganism with others, dealing with difficult scenarios with non-vegans etc)

_____
_____
_____
_____
_____
_____
_____

MY DAILY VEGAN DIARY

Day 87:

How did my day go?

_____
_____
_____
_____
_____
_____
_____
_____
_____
_____
_____
_____
_____
_____
_____
_____
_____
_____
_____
_____
_____
_____
_____
_____
_____
_____
_____
_____
_____

Has my food intake been sufficient in:

Protein ☐   Calcium ☐   Iron ☐   Omega 3 ☐   Vitamin C ☐   Fibre ☐

Notes

How has my mood been today?

_____

_____

_____

_____

_____

_____

Is there anything I would do differently the following days?

(This could be in regard to your food intake, your discussions about veganism with others, dealing with difficult scenarios with non-vegans etc)

_____

_____

_____

_____

_____

_____

_____

MY DAILY VEGAN DIARY

Day 88: _____

How did my day go?

_____
_____
_____
_____
_____
_____
_____
_____
_____
_____
_____
_____
_____
_____
_____
_____
_____
_____
_____
_____
_____
_____
_____
_____
_____
_____
_____
_____

Has my food intake been sufficient in:

Protein ☐   Calcium ☐   Iron ☐   Omega 3 ☐   Vitamin C ☐   Fibre ☐

Notes

How has my mood been today?

_____
_____
_____
_____
_____
_____

Is there anything I would do differently the following days?

(This could be in regard to your food intake, your discussions about
veganism with others, dealing with difficult scenarios with non-vegans
etc)

_____
_____
_____
_____
_____
_____
_____

MY DAILY VEGAN DIARY

Day 89

How did my day go?

_____
_____
_____
_____
_____
_____
_____
_____
_____
_____
_____
_____
_____
_____
_____
_____
_____
_____
_____
_____
_____
_____
_____
_____
_____
_____
_____
_____

Has my food intake been sufficient in:

Protein ☐   Calcium ☐   Iron ☐   Omega 3 ☐   Vitamin C ☐   Fibre ☐

Notes

How has my mood been today?

_____

_____

_____

_____

_____

_____

Is there anything I would do differently the following days?
(This could be in regard to your food intake, your discussions about veganism with others, dealing with difficult scenarios with non-vegans etc)

_____

_____

_____

_____

_____

_____

_____

MY DAILY VEGAN DIARY

Day 90.

How did my day go?

_____
_____
_____
_____
_____
_____
_____
_____
_____
_____
_____
_____
_____
_____
_____
_____
_____
_____
_____
_____
_____
_____
_____
_____
_____

Has my food intake been sufficient in:

Protein ☐   Calcium ☐   Iron ☐   Omega 3 ☐   Vitamin C ☐   Fibre ☐

Notes

How has my mood been today?

_____

_____

_____

_____

_____

_____

Is there anything I would do differently the following days?

(This could be in regard to your food intake, your discussions about

veganism with others, dealing with difficult scenarios with non-vegans

etc)

_____

_____

_____

_____

_____

_____

_____

MY DAILY VEGAN DIARY

Day 91: _____

How did my day go?

_____
_____
_____
_____
_____
_____
_____
_____
_____
_____
_____
_____
_____
_____
_____
_____
_____
_____
_____
_____
_____
_____
_____
_____
_____
_____
_____

Has my food intake been sufficient in:

Protein ☐   Calcium ☐   Iron ☐   Omega 3 ☐   Vitamin C ☐   Fibre ☐

Notes

How has my mood been today?

_____

_____

_____

_____

_____

_____

Is there anything I would do differently the following days?

(This could be in regard to your food intake, your discussions about

veganism with others, dealing with difficult scenarios with non-vegans

etc)

_____

_____

_____

_____

_____

_____

_____

MY DAILY VEGAN DIARY

Day 92.

How did my day go?

_____
_____
_____
_____
_____
_____
_____
_____
_____
_____
_____
_____
_____
_____
_____
_____
_____
_____
_____
_____
_____
_____
_____
_____
_____
_____
_____

Has my food intake been sufficient in:

Protein ☐   Calcium ☐   Iron ☐   Omega 3 ☐   Vitamin C ☐   Fibre ☐

Notes

How has my mood been today?

_____

_____

_____

_____

_____

_____

Is there anything I would do differently the following days?

(This could be in regard to your food intake, your discussions about

veganism with others, dealing with difficult scenarios with non-vegans

etc)

_____

_____

_____

_____

_____

_____

_____

MY DAILY VEGAN DIARY

Day 93: _____

How did my day go?

_____
_____
_____
_____
_____
_____
_____
_____
_____
_____
_____
_____
_____
_____
_____
_____
_____
_____
_____
_____
_____
_____
_____
_____
_____
_____
_____
_____
_____

Has my food intake been sufficient in:

Protein ☐   Calcium ☐   Iron ☐   Omega 3 ☐   Vitamin C ☐   Fibre ☐

Notes

How has my mood been today?

_____

_____

_____

_____

_____

Is there anything I would do differently the following days?

(This could be in regard to your food intake, your discussions about veganism with others, dealing with difficult scenarios with non-vegans etc)

_____

_____

_____

_____

_____

_____

_____

MY DAILY VEGAN DIARY

Day 94: _____

How did my day go?

_____
_____
_____
_____
_____
_____
_____
_____
_____
_____
_____
_____
_____
_____
_____
_____
_____
_____
_____
_____
_____
_____
_____
_____
_____
_____
_____

Has my food intake been sufficient in:

Protein ☐   Calcium ☐   Iron ☐   Omega 3 ☐   Vitamin C ☐   Fibre ☐

Notes

How has my mood been today?

Is there anything I would do differently the following days?
(This could be in regard to your food intake, your discussions about veganism with others, dealing with difficult scenarios with non-vegans etc)

MY DAILY VEGAN DIARY

Day 95

How did my day go?

_____
_____
_____
_____
_____
_____
_____
_____
_____
_____
_____
_____
_____
_____
_____
_____
_____
_____
_____
_____
_____
_____
_____
_____
_____
_____
_____
_____
_____

Has my food intake been sufficient in:

Protein ☐   Calcium ☐   Iron ☐   Omega 3 ☐   Vitamin C ☐   Fibre ☐

Notes

How has my mood been today?

_____

_____

_____

_____

_____

_____

Is there anything I would do differently the following days?

(This could be in regard to your food intake, your discussions about veganism with others, dealing with difficult scenarios with non-vegans etc)

_____

_____

_____

_____

_____

_____

_____

MY DAILY VEGAN DIARY

Day 96: _____

How did my day go?

_____
_____
_____
_____
_____
_____
_____
_____
_____
_____
_____
_____
_____
_____
_____
_____
_____
_____
_____
_____
_____
_____
_____
_____
_____
_____
_____
_____
_____

Has my food intake been sufficient in:

Protein ☐   Calcium ☐   Iron ☐   Omega 3 ☐   Vitamin C ☐   Fibre ☐

Notes

How has my mood been today?

_____

_____

_____

_____

_____

Is there anything I would do differently the following days?

(This could be in regard to your food intake, your discussions about

veganism with others, dealing with difficult scenarios with non-vegans

etc)

_____

_____

_____

_____

_____

_____

_____

MY DAILY VEGAN DIARY

Day 97: _____

How did my day go?

_____
_____
_____
_____
_____
_____
_____
_____
_____
_____
_____
_____
_____
_____
_____
_____
_____
_____
_____
_____
_____
_____
_____
_____
_____

Has my food intake been sufficient in:

Protein ☐   Calcium ☐   Iron ☐   Omega 3 ☐   Vitamin C ☐   Fibre ☐

Notes

How has my mood been today?

_____

_____

_____

_____

_____

_____

Is there anything I would do differently the following days?

(This could be in regard to your food intake, your discussions about

veganism with others, dealing with difficult scenarios with non-vegans

etc)

_____

_____

_____

_____

_____

_____

_____

MY DAILY VEGAN DIARY

Day 98: _____

How did my day go?

_____
_____
_____
_____
_____
_____
_____
_____
_____
_____
_____
_____
_____
_____
_____
_____
_____
_____
_____
_____
_____
_____
_____
_____
_____
_____
_____
_____

Has my food intake been sufficient in:

Protein ☐   Calcium ☐   Iron ☐   Omega 3 ☐   Vitamin C ☐   Fibre ☐

Notes

How has my mood been today?

Is there anything I would do differently the following days?
(This could be in regard to your food intake, your discussions about
veganism with others, dealing with difficult scenarios with non-vegans
etc)

MY DAILY VEGAN DIARY

Day 99: _____

How did my day go?

_____
_____
_____
_____
_____
_____
_____
_____
_____
_____
_____
_____
_____
_____
_____
_____
_____
_____
_____
_____
_____
_____
_____
_____
_____
_____
_____
_____
_____

Has my food intake been sufficient in:

Protein ☐   Calcium ☐   Iron ☐   Omega 3 ☐   Vitamin C ☐   Fibre ☐

Notes

How has my mood been today?

_____

_____

_____

_____

_____

_____

Is there anything I would do differently the following days?

(This could be in regard to your food intake, your discussions about veganism with others, dealing with difficult scenarios with non-vegans etc)

_____

_____

_____

_____

_____

_____

_____

MY DAILY VEGAN DIARY

Day 100: _____

How did my day go?

_____
_____
_____
_____
_____
_____
_____
_____
_____
_____
_____
_____
_____
_____
_____
_____
_____
_____
_____
_____
_____
_____
_____
_____
_____
_____
_____
_____

Has my food intake been sufficient in:

Protein ☐   Calcium ☐   Iron ☐   Omega 3 ☐   Vitamin C ☐   Fibre ☐

Notes

How has my mood been today?

_____
_____
_____
_____
_____
_____

Is there anything I would do differently the following days?

(This could be in regard to your food intake, your discussions about veganism with others, dealing with difficult scenarios with non-vegans etc)

_____
_____
_____
_____
_____
_____

MY DAILY VEGAN DIARY

Day 101.

How did my day go?

_____
_____
_____
_____
_____
_____
_____
_____
_____
_____
_____
_____
_____
_____
_____
_____
_____
_____
_____
_____
_____
_____
_____
_____
_____
_____
_____
_____

Has my food intake been sufficient in:

Protein ☐   Calcium ☐   Iron ☐   Omega 3 ☐   Vitamin C ☐   Fibre ☐

Notes

How has my mood been today?

_____
_____
_____
_____
_____
_____

Is there anything I would do differently the following days?
(This could be in regard to your food intake, your discussions about veganism with others, dealing with difficult scenarios with non-vegans etc)

_____
_____
_____
_____
_____
_____
_____

MY DAILY VEGAN DIARY

Day 102: _____

How did my day go?

_____
_____
_____
_____
_____
_____
_____
_____
_____
_____
_____
_____
_____
_____
_____
_____
_____
_____
_____
_____
_____
_____
_____
_____
_____
_____
_____
_____
_____
_____
_____

Has my food intake been sufficient in:

Protein ☐   Calcium ☐   Iron ☐   Omega 3 ☐   Vitamin C ☐   Fibre ☐

Notes

How has my mood been today?

_____

_____

_____

_____

_____

_____

Is there anything I would do differently the following days?

(This could be in regard to your food intake, your discussions about

veganism with others, dealing with difficult scenarios with non-vegans

etc)

_____

_____

_____

_____

_____

_____

_____

MY DAILY VEGAN DIARY

Day 103: _____

How did my day go?

_____
_____
_____
_____
_____
_____
_____
_____
_____
_____
_____
_____
_____
_____
_____
_____
_____
_____
_____
_____
_____
_____
_____
_____
_____
_____
_____

Has my food intake been sufficient in:

Protein ☐   Calcium ☐   Iron ☐   Omega 3 ☐   Vitamin C ☐   Fibre ☐

Notes

How has my mood been today?

_____

_____

_____

_____

_____

_____

Is there anything I would do differently the following days?

(This could be in regard to your food intake, your discussions about

veganism with others, dealing with difficult scenarios with non-vegans

etc)

_____

_____

_____

_____

_____

_____

_____

MY DAILY VEGAN DIARY

Day 104: _____

How did my day go?

_____
_____
_____
_____
_____
_____
_____
_____
_____
_____
_____
_____
_____
_____
_____
_____
_____
_____
_____
_____
_____
_____
_____
_____
_____
_____
_____

Has my food intake been sufficient in:

Protein ☐   Calcium ☐   Iron ☐   Omega 3 ☐   Vitamin C ☐   Fibre ☐

Notes

How has my mood been today?

_____

_____

_____

_____

_____

Is there anything I would do differently the following days?

(This could be in regard to your food intake, your discussions about veganism with others, dealing with difficult scenarios with non-vegans etc)

_____

_____

_____

_____

_____

_____

_____

MY DAILY VEGAN DIARY

Day 105: _____

How did my day go?

_____
_____
_____
_____
_____
_____
_____
_____
_____
_____
_____
_____
_____
_____
_____
_____
_____
_____
_____
_____
_____
_____
_____
_____
_____
_____
_____
_____
_____
_____

Has my food intake been sufficient in:

Protein ☐   Calcium ☐   Iron ☐   Omega 3 ☐   Vitamin C ☐   Fibre ☐

Notes

How has my mood been today?

_____

_____

_____

_____

_____

_____

Is there anything I would do differently the following days?

(This could be in regard to your food intake, your discussions about veganism with others, dealing with difficult scenarios with non-vegans etc)

_____

_____

_____

_____

_____

_____

_____

MY DAILY VEGAN DIARY

Day 106: _____

How did my day go?

_____
_____
_____
_____
_____
_____
_____
_____
_____
_____
_____
_____
_____
_____
_____
_____
_____
_____
_____
_____
_____
_____
_____
_____
_____
_____
_____
_____
_____

Has my food intake been sufficient in:

Protein ☐   Calcium ☐   Iron ☐   Omega 3 ☐   Vitamin C ☐   Fibre ☐

Notes

How has my mood been today?

_____

_____

_____

_____

_____

_____

Is there anything I would do differently the following days?

(This could be in regard to your food intake, your discussions about

veganism with others, dealing with difficult scenarios with non-vegans

etc)

_____

_____

_____

_____

_____

_____

_____

MY DAILY VEGAN DIARY

Day 107: _____

How did my day go?

_____
_____
_____
_____
_____
_____
_____
_____
_____
_____
_____
_____
_____
_____
_____
_____
_____
_____
_____
_____
_____
_____
_____
_____
_____
_____
_____
_____

Has my food intake been sufficient in:

Protein ☐   Calcium ☐   Iron ☐   Omega 3 ☐   Vitamin C ☐   Fibre ☐

Notes

How has my mood been today?

_____
_____
_____
_____
_____
_____

Is there anything I would do differently the following days?
(This could be in regard to your food intake, your discussions about veganism with others, dealing with difficult scenarios with non-vegans etc)

_____
_____
_____
_____
_____
_____
_____

MY DAILY VEGAN DIARY

Day 108: _____

How did my day go?

_____
_____
_____
_____
_____
_____
_____
_____
_____
_____
_____
_____
_____
_____
_____
_____
_____
_____
_____
_____
_____
_____
_____
_____
_____
_____
_____
_____
_____

Has my food intake been sufficient in:

Protein ☐   Calcium ☐   Iron ☐   Omega 3 ☐   Vitamin C ☐   Fibre ☐

Notes

How has my mood been today?

_____

_____

_____

_____

_____

_____

Is there anything I would do differently the following days?

(This could be in regard to your food intake, your discussions about veganism with others, dealing with difficult scenarios with non-vegans etc)

_____

_____

_____

_____

_____

_____

_____

MY DAILY VEGAN DIARY

Day 109:

How did my day go?

_____
_____
_____
_____
_____
_____
_____
_____
_____
_____
_____
_____
_____
_____
_____
_____
_____
_____
_____
_____
_____
_____
_____
_____
_____
_____
_____
_____
_____
_____
_____

Has my food intake been sufficient in:

Protein ☐　　Calcium ☐　　Iron ☐　　Omega 3 ☐　　Vitamin C ☐　　Fibre ☐

Notes

How has my mood been today?

_____
_____
_____
_____
_____
_____

Is there anything I would do differently the following days?
(This could be in regard to your food intake, your discussions about veganism with others, dealing with difficult scenarios with non-vegans etc)

_____
_____
_____
_____
_____
_____
_____

MY DAILY VEGAN DIARY

Day 110: _____

How did my day go?

_____
_____
_____
_____
_____
_____
_____
_____
_____
_____
_____
_____
_____
_____
_____
_____
_____
_____
_____
_____
_____
_____
_____
_____
_____
_____
_____

Has my food intake been sufficient in:

Protein ☐   Calcium ☐   Iron ☐   Omega 3 ☐   Vitamin C ☐   Fibre ☐

Notes

How has my mood been today?

_____

_____

_____

_____

_____

_____

Is there anything I would do differently the following days?

(This could be in regard to your food intake, your discussions about

veganism with others, dealing with difficult scenarios with non-vegans

etc)

_____

_____

_____

_____

_____

_____

_____

MY DAILY VEGAN DIARY

Day 111: _____

How did my day go?

_____
_____
_____
_____
_____
_____
_____
_____
_____
_____
_____
_____
_____
_____
_____
_____
_____
_____
_____
_____
_____
_____
_____
_____
_____
_____
_____

Has my food intake been sufficient in:

Protein ☐   Calcium ☐   Iron ☐   Omega 3 ☐   Vitamin C ☐   Fibre ☐

Notes

How has my mood been today?

_____

_____

_____

_____

_____

_____

Is there anything I would do differently the following days?

(This could be in regard to your food intake, your discussions about veganism with others, dealing with difficult scenarios with non-vegans etc)

_____

_____

_____

_____

_____

_____

_____

MY DAILY VEGAN DIARY

Day 112: _____

How did my day go?

_____
_____
_____
_____
_____
_____
_____
_____
_____
_____
_____
_____
_____
_____
_____
_____
_____
_____
_____
_____
_____
_____
_____
_____
_____
_____
_____
_____

Has my food intake been sufficient in:

Protein ☐   Calcium ☐   Iron ☐   Omega 3 ☐   Vitamin C ☐   Fibre ☐

Notes

How has my mood been today?

_____

_____

_____

_____

_____

_____

Is there anything I would do differently the following days?
(This could be in regard to your food intake, your discussions about veganism with others, dealing with difficult scenarios with non-vegans etc)

_____

_____

_____

_____

_____

_____

_____

MY DAILY VEGAN DIARY

Day 113: _____

How did my day go?

_____
_____
_____
_____
_____
_____
_____
_____
_____
_____
_____
_____
_____
_____
_____
_____
_____
_____
_____
_____
_____
_____
_____
_____
_____
_____
_____
_____

Has my food intake been sufficient in:

Protein ☐   Calcium ☐   Iron ☐   Omega 3 ☐   Vitamin C ☐   Fibre ☐

Notes

How has my mood been today?

_____
_____
_____
_____
_____
_____

Is there anything I would do differently the following days?
(This could be in regard to your food intake, your discussions about veganism with others, dealing with difficult scenarios with non-vegans etc)

_____
_____
_____
_____
_____
_____
_____

MY DAILY VEGAN DIARY

Day 114: _____

How did my day go?

_____
_____
_____
_____
_____
_____
_____
_____
_____
_____
_____
_____
_____
_____
_____
_____
_____
_____
_____
_____
_____
_____
_____
_____
_____
_____
_____
_____

Has my food intake been sufficient in:

Protein ☐   Calcium ☐   Iron ☐   Omega 3 ☐   Vitamin C ☐   Fibre ☐

Notes

How has my mood been today?

_____

_____

_____

_____

_____

_____

Is there anything I would do differently the following days?

(This could be in regard to your food intake, your discussions about

veganism with others, dealing with difficult scenarios with non-vegans

etc)

_____

_____

_____

_____

_____

_____

_____

MY DAILY VEGAN DIARY

Day 115: _____

How did my day go?

_____
_____
_____
_____
_____
_____
_____
_____
_____
_____
_____
_____
_____
_____
_____
_____
_____
_____
_____
_____
_____
_____
_____
_____
_____
_____
_____
_____
_____

Has my food intake been sufficient in:

Protein ☐   Calcium ☐   Iron ☐   Omega 3 ☐   Vitamin C ☐   Fibre ☐

Notes

How has my mood been today?

Is there anything I would do differently the following days?
(This could be in regard to your food intake, your discussions about veganism with others, dealing with difficult scenarios with non-vegans etc)

MY DAILY VEGAN DIARY

Day 116: _____

How did my day go?

_____
_____
_____
_____
_____
_____
_____
_____
_____
_____
_____
_____
_____
_____
_____
_____
_____
_____
_____
_____
_____
_____
_____
_____
_____
_____
_____
_____
_____

Has my food intake been sufficient in:

Protein ☐   Calcium ☐   Iron ☐   Omega 3 ☐   Vitamin C ☐   Fibre ☐

Notes

How has my mood been today?

_____

_____

_____

_____

_____

_____

Is there anything I would do differently the following days?

(This could be in regard to your food intake, your discussions about veganism with others, dealing with difficult scenarios with non-vegans etc)

_____

_____

_____

_____

_____

_____

_____

MY DAILY VEGAN DIARY

Day 117: _____

How did my day go?

_____
_____
_____
_____
_____
_____
_____
_____
_____
_____
_____
_____
_____
_____
_____
_____
_____
_____
_____
_____
_____
_____
_____
_____
_____

Has my food intake been sufficient in:

Protein ☐   Calcium ☐   Iron ☐   Omega 3 ☐   Vitamin C ☐   Fibre ☐

Notes

How has my mood been today?

_____

_____

_____

_____

_____

_____

Is there anything I would do differently the following days?

(This could be in regard to your food intake, your discussions about veganism with others, dealing with difficult scenarios with non-vegans etc)

_____

_____

_____

_____

_____

_____

_____

MY DAILY VEGAN DIARY

Day 118: _____

How did my day go?

_____
_____
_____
_____
_____
_____
_____
_____
_____
_____
_____
_____
_____
_____
_____
_____
_____
_____
_____
_____
_____
_____
_____
_____
_____
_____
_____
_____

Has my food intake been sufficient in:

Protein ☐   Calcium ☐   Iron ☐   Omega 3 ☐   Vitamin C ☐   Fibre ☐

Notes

How has my mood been today?

Is there anything I would do differently the following days?
(This could be in regard to your food intake, your discussions about veganism with others, dealing with difficult scenarios with non-vegans etc)

MY DAILY VEGAN DIARY

Day 119: _____

How did my day go?

_____
_____
_____
_____
_____
_____
_____
_____
_____
_____
_____
_____
_____
_____
_____
_____
_____
_____
_____
_____
_____
_____
_____
_____
_____
_____

Has my food intake been sufficient in:

Protein ☐   Calcium ☐   Iron ☐   Omega 3 ☐   Vitamin C ☐   Fibre ☐

Notes

How has my mood been today?

_____

_____

_____

_____

_____

_____

Is there anything I would do differently the following days?

(This could be in regard to your food intake, your discussions about veganism with others, dealing with difficult scenarios with non-vegans etc)

_____

_____

_____

_____

_____

_____

_____

MY DAILY VEGAN DIARY

Day 120: _____

How did my day go?

_____
_____
_____
_____
_____
_____
_____
_____
_____
_____
_____
_____
_____
_____
_____
_____
_____
_____
_____
_____
_____
_____
_____
_____
_____
_____

Has my food intake been sufficient in:

Protein ☐   Calcium ☐   Iron ☐   Omega 3 ☐   Vitamin C ☐   Fibre ☐

Notes

How has my mood been today?

_____

_____

_____

_____

_____

_____

Is there anything I would do differently the following days?

(This could be in regard to your food intake, your discussions about veganism with others, dealing with difficult scenarios with non-vegans etc)

_____

_____

_____

_____

_____

_____

_____

MY DAILY VEGAN DIARY

Day 121: _____

How did my day go?

_____
_____
_____
_____
_____
_____
_____
_____
_____
_____
_____
_____
_____
_____
_____
_____
_____
_____
_____
_____
_____
_____
_____
_____
_____
_____
_____

Has my food intake been sufficient in:

Protein ☐   Calcium ☐   Iron ☐   Omega 3 ☐   Vitamin C ☐   Fibre ☐

Notes

How has my mood been today?

_____
_____
_____
_____
_____
_____

Is there anything I would do differently the following days?
(This could be in regard to your food intake, your discussions about veganism with others, dealing with difficult scenarios with non-vegans etc)

_____
_____
_____
_____
_____
_____
_____

MY DAILY VEGAN DIARY

Day 122: _____

How did my day go?

_____
_____
_____
_____
_____
_____
_____
_____
_____
_____
_____
_____
_____
_____
_____
_____
_____
_____
_____
_____
_____
_____
_____
_____
_____
_____
_____
_____
_____

Has my food intake been sufficient in:

Protein ☐ Calcium ☐ Iron ☐ Omega 3 ☐ Vitamin C ☐ Fibre ☐

Notes

How has my mood been today?

_____
_____
_____
_____
_____
_____

Is there anything I would do differently the following days?
(This could be in regard to your food intake, your discussions about veganism with others, dealing with difficult scenarios with non-vegans etc)

_____
_____
_____
_____
_____
_____
_____

MY DAILY VEGAN DIARY

Day 123. _____

How did my day go?

_____
_____
_____
_____
_____
_____
_____
_____
_____
_____
_____
_____
_____
_____
_____
_____
_____
_____
_____
_____
_____
_____
_____
_____
_____
_____
_____
_____
_____
_____

Has my food intake been sufficient in:

Protein ☐   Calcium ☐   Iron ☐   Omega 3 ☐   Vitamin C ☐   Fibre ☐

Notes

How has my mood been today?

_____

_____

_____

_____

_____

_____

Is there anything I would do differently the following days?

(This could be in regard to your food intake, your discussions about veganism with others, dealing with difficult scenarios with non-vegans etc)

_____

_____

_____

_____

_____

_____

MY DAILY VEGAN DIARY

Day 124: _____

How did my day go?

_____
_____
_____
_____
_____
_____
_____
_____
_____
_____
_____
_____
_____
_____
_____
_____
_____
_____
_____
_____
_____
_____
_____
_____
_____
_____
_____

Has my food intake been sufficient in:

Protein ☐   Calcium ☐   Iron ☐   Omega 3 ☐   Vitamin C ☐   Fibre ☐

Notes

How has my mood been today?

_____
_____
_____
_____
_____
_____

Is there anything I would do differently the following days?
(This could be in regard to your food intake, your discussions about
veganism with others, dealing with difficult scenarios with non-vegans
etc)

_____
_____
_____
_____
_____
_____
_____

MY DAILY VEGAN DIARY

Day 125.

How did my day go?

_____
_____
_____
_____
_____
_____
_____
_____
_____
_____
_____
_____
_____
_____
_____
_____
_____
_____
_____
_____
_____
_____
_____
_____
_____
_____

Has my food intake been sufficient in:

Protein ☐   Calcium ☐   Iron ☐   Omega 3 ☐   Vitamin C ☐   Fibre ☐

Notes

How has my mood been today?

_____

_____

_____

_____

_____

_____

Is there anything I would do differently the following days?
(This could be in regard to your food intake, your discussions about veganism with others, dealing with difficult scenarios with non-vegans etc)

_____

_____

_____

_____

_____

_____

_____

MY DAILY VEGAN DIARY

Day 126: _____

How did my day go?

_____
_____
_____
_____
_____
_____
_____
_____
_____
_____
_____
_____
_____
_____
_____
_____
_____
_____
_____
_____
_____
_____
_____
_____
_____
_____

Has my food intake been sufficient in:

Protein ☐   Calcium ☐   Iron ☐   Omega 3 ☐   Vitamin C ☐   Fibre ☐

Notes

How has my mood been today?

_____

_____

_____

_____

_____

_____

Is there anything I would do differently the following days?
(This could be in regard to your food intake, your discussions about
veganism with others, dealing with difficult scenarios with non-vegans
etc)

_____

_____

_____

_____

_____

_____

_____

MY DAILY VEGAN DIARY

Day 127: _____

How did my day go?

_____
_____
_____
_____
_____
_____
_____
_____
_____
_____
_____
_____
_____
_____
_____
_____
_____
_____
_____
_____
_____
_____
_____
_____
_____
_____
_____
_____
_____

Has my food intake been sufficient in:

Protein ☐   Calcium ☐   Iron ☐   Omega 3 ☐   Vitamin C ☐   Fibre ☐

Notes

How has my mood been today?

_____
_____
_____
_____
_____
_____

Is there anything I would do differently the following days?
(This could be in regard to your food intake, your discussions about veganism with others, dealing with difficult scenarios with non-vegans etc)

_____
_____
_____
_____
_____
_____
_____

MY DAILY VEGAN DIARY

Day 128: _____

How did my day go?

_____
_____
_____
_____
_____
_____
_____
_____
_____
_____
_____
_____
_____
_____
_____
_____
_____
_____
_____
_____
_____
_____
_____
_____
_____
_____
_____
_____
_____

Has my food intake been sufficient in:

Protein ☐   Calcium ☐   Iron ☐   Omega 3 ☐   Vitamin C ☐   Fibre ☐

Notes

How has my mood been today?

_____

_____

_____

_____

_____

_____

Is there anything I would do differently the following days?

(This could be in regard to your food intake, your discussions about veganism with others, dealing with difficult scenarios with non-vegans etc)

_____

_____

_____

_____

_____

_____

_____

MY DAILY VEGAN DIARY

Day 129:

How did my day go?

_____
_____
_____
_____
_____
_____
_____
_____
_____
_____
_____
_____
_____
_____
_____
_____
_____
_____
_____
_____
_____
_____
_____
_____
_____

Has my food intake been sufficient in:

Protein ☐   Calcium ☐   Iron ☐   Omega 3 ☐   Vitamin C ☐   Fibre ☐

Notes

How has my mood been today?

_____

_____

_____

_____

_____

_____

Is there anything I would do differently the following days?

(This could be in regard to your food intake, your discussions about veganism with others, dealing with difficult scenarios with non-vegans etc)

_____

_____

_____

_____

_____

_____

_____

MY DAILY VEGAN DIARY

Day 130:

How did my day go?

_____
_____
_____
_____
_____
_____
_____
_____
_____
_____
_____
_____
_____
_____
_____
_____
_____
_____
_____
_____
_____
_____
_____
_____
_____
_____

Has my food intake been sufficient in:

Protein ☐   Calcium ☐   Iron ☐   Omega 3 ☐   Vitamin C ☐   Fibre ☐

Notes

How has my mood been today?

_____

_____

_____

_____

_____

Is there anything I would do differently the following days?

(This could be in regard to your food intake, your discussions about veganism with others, dealing with difficult scenarios with non-vegans etc)

_____

_____

_____

_____

_____

_____

MY DAILY VEGAN DIARY

Day 131:

How did my day go?

_____
_____
_____
_____
_____
_____
_____
_____
_____
_____
_____
_____
_____
_____
_____
_____
_____
_____
_____
_____
_____
_____
_____
_____
_____
_____
_____
_____

Has my food intake been sufficient in:

Protein ☐   Calcium ☐   Iron ☐   Omega 3 ☐   Vitamin C ☐   Fibre ☐

Notes

How has my mood been today?

_____
_____
_____
_____
_____
_____

Is there anything I would do differently the following days?
(This could be in regard to your food intake, your discussions about veganism with others, dealing with difficult scenarios with non-vegans etc)

_____
_____
_____
_____
_____
_____
_____

MY DAILY VEGAN DIARY

Day 132. _____

How did my day go?

_____
_____
_____
_____
_____
_____
_____
_____
_____
_____
_____
_____
_____
_____
_____
_____
_____
_____
_____
_____
_____
_____
_____
_____
_____
_____
_____
_____
_____

Has my food intake been sufficient in:

Protein ☐   Calcium ☐   Iron ☐   Omega 3 ☐   Vitamin C ☐   Fibre ☐

Notes

How has my mood been today?

_____

_____

_____

_____

_____

_____

Is there anything I would do differently the following days?

(This could be in regard to your food intake, your discussions about veganism with others, dealing with difficult scenarios with non-vegans etc)

_____

_____

_____

_____

_____

_____

_____

MY DAILY VEGAN DIARY

Day 133: _____

How did my day go?

_____
_____
_____
_____
_____
_____
_____
_____
_____
_____
_____
_____
_____
_____
_____
_____
_____
_____
_____
_____
_____
_____
_____
_____
_____

Has my food intake been sufficient in:

Protein ☐   Calcium ☐   Iron ☐   Omega 3 ☐   Vitamin C ☐   Fibre ☐

Notes

How has my mood been today?

_____
_____
_____
_____
_____
_____

Is there anything I would do differently the following days?
(This could be in regard to your food intake, your discussions about veganism with others, dealing with difficult scenarios with non-vegans etc)

_____
_____
_____
_____
_____
_____
_____

MY DAILY VEGAN DIARY

Day 134:

How did my day go?

_____
_____
_____
_____
_____
_____
_____
_____
_____
_____
_____
_____
_____
_____
_____
_____
_____
_____
_____
_____
_____
_____
_____
_____
_____
_____

Has my food intake been sufficient in:

Protein ☐   Calcium ☐   Iron ☐   Omega 3 ☐   Vitamin C ☐   Fibre ☐

Notes

How has my mood been today?

_____

_____

_____

_____

_____

_____

Is there anything I would do differently the following days?

(This could be in regard to your food intake, your discussions about veganism with others, dealing with difficult scenarios with non-vegans etc)

_____

_____

_____

_____

_____

_____

_____

MY DAILY VEGAN DIARY

Day 135:

How did my day go?

_____
_____
_____
_____
_____
_____
_____
_____
_____
_____
_____
_____
_____
_____
_____
_____
_____
_____
_____
_____
_____
_____
_____
_____
_____

Has my food intake been sufficient in:

Protein ☐   Calcium ☐   Iron ☐   Omega 3 ☐   Vitamin C ☐   Fibre ☐

Notes

How has my mood been today?

_____

_____

_____

_____

_____

_____

Is there anything I would do differently the following days?

(This could be in regard to your food intake, your discussions about veganism with others, dealing with difficult scenarios with non-vegans etc)

_____

_____

_____

_____

_____

_____

_____

MY DAILY VEGAN DIARY

Day 136: _____

How did my day go?

_____
_____
_____
_____
_____
_____
_____
_____
_____
_____
_____
_____
_____
_____
_____
_____
_____
_____
_____
_____
_____
_____
_____
_____
_____
_____

Has my food intake been sufficient in:

Protein ☐   Calcium ☐   Iron ☐   Omega 3 ☐   Vitamin C ☐   Fibre ☐

Notes

How has my mood been today?

_____

_____

_____

_____

_____

_____

Is there anything I would do differently the following days?
(This could be in regard to your food intake, your discussions about veganism with others, dealing with difficult scenarios with non-vegans etc)

_____

_____

_____

_____

_____

_____

_____

MY DAILY VEGAN DIARY

Day 137: _____

How did my day go?

_____
_____
_____
_____
_____
_____
_____
_____
_____
_____
_____
_____
_____
_____
_____
_____
_____
_____
_____
_____
_____
_____
_____
_____
_____

Has my food intake been sufficient in:

Protein ☐   Calcium ☐   Iron ☐   Omega 3 ☐   Vitamin C ☐   Fibre ☐

Notes

How has my mood been today?

_____

_____

_____

_____

_____

_____

Is there anything I would do differently the following days?

(This could be in regard to your food intake, your discussions about veganism with others, dealing with difficult scenarios with non-vegans etc)

_____

_____

_____

_____

_____

_____

_____

MY DAILY VEGAN DIARY

Day 138: _____

How did my day go?

_____
_____
_____
_____
_____
_____
_____
_____
_____
_____
_____
_____
_____
_____
_____
_____
_____
_____
_____
_____
_____
_____
_____
_____
_____
_____
_____
_____
_____

Has my food intake been sufficient in:

Protein ☐   Calcium ☐   Iron ☐   Omega 3 ☐   Vitamin C ☐   Fibre ☐

Notes

How has my mood been today?

Is there anything I would do differently the following days?
(This could be in regard to your food intake, your discussions about veganism with others, dealing with difficult scenarios with non-vegans etc)

MY DAILY VEGAN DIARY

Day 139: _____

How did my day go?

_____
_____
_____
_____
_____
_____
_____
_____
_____
_____
_____
_____
_____
_____
_____
_____
_____
_____
_____
_____
_____
_____
_____
_____
_____
_____
_____

Has my food intake been sufficient in:

Protein ☐   Calcium ☐   Iron ☐   Omega 3 ☐   Vitamin C ☐   Fibre ☐

Notes

How has my mood been today?

_____
_____
_____
_____
_____
_____

Is there anything I would do differently the following days?
(This could be in regard to your food intake, your discussions about veganism with others, dealing with difficult scenarios with non-vegans etc)

_____
_____
_____
_____
_____
_____
_____

MY DAILY VEGAN DIARY

Day 140: _____

How did my day go?

_____
_____
_____
_____
_____
_____
_____
_____
_____
_____
_____
_____
_____
_____
_____
_____
_____
_____
_____
_____
_____
_____
_____
_____
_____
_____
_____
_____

Has my food intake been sufficient in:

Protein ☐   Calcium ☐   Iron ☐   Omega 3 ☐   Vitamin C ☐   Fibre ☐

Notes

How has my mood been today?

_____

_____

_____

_____

_____

_____

Is there anything I would do differently the following days?

(This could be in regard to your food intake, your discussions about veganism with others, dealing with difficult scenarios with non-vegans etc)

_____

_____

_____

_____

_____

_____

_____

MY DAILY VEGAN DIARY

Day 141:

How did my day go?

_____
_____
_____
_____
_____
_____
_____
_____
_____
_____
_____
_____
_____
_____
_____
_____
_____
_____
_____
_____
_____
_____
_____
_____
_____
_____
_____

Has my food intake been sufficient in:

Protein ☐   Calcium ☐   Iron ☐   Omega 3 ☐   Vitamin C ☐   Fibre ☐

Notes

How has my mood been today?

_____
_____
_____
_____
_____
_____

Is there anything I would do differently the following days?

(This could be in regard to your food intake, your discussions about veganism with others, dealing with difficult scenarios with non-vegans etc)

_____
_____
_____
_____
_____
_____
_____

MY DAILY VEGAN DIARY

Day 142: _____

How did my day go?

_____
_____
_____
_____
_____
_____
_____
_____
_____
_____
_____
_____
_____
_____
_____
_____
_____
_____
_____
_____
_____
_____
_____
_____

Has my food intake been sufficient in:

Protein ☐   Calcium ☐   Iron ☐   Omega 3 ☐   Vitamin C ☐   Fibre ☐

Notes

How has my mood been today?

_____
_____
_____
_____
_____
_____

Is there anything I would do differently the following days?
(This could be in regard to your food intake, your discussions about
veganism with others, dealing with difficult scenarios with non-vegans
etc)

_____
_____
_____
_____
_____
_____
_____

MY DAILY VEGAN DIARY

Day 143:

How did my day go?

_____
_____
_____
_____
_____
_____
_____
_____
_____
_____
_____
_____
_____
_____
_____
_____
_____
_____
_____
_____
_____
_____
_____
_____
_____
_____
_____
_____

Has my food intake been sufficient in:

Protein ☐   Calcium ☐   Iron ☐   Omega 3 ☐   Vitamin C ☐   Fibre ☐

Notes

How has my mood been today?

_____
_____
_____
_____
_____
_____

Is there anything I would do differently the following days?
(This could be in regard to your food intake, your discussions about veganism with others, dealing with difficult scenarios with non-vegans etc)

_____
_____
_____
_____
_____
_____
_____

MY DAILY VEGAN DIARY

Day 144: _____

How did my day go?

_____
_____
_____
_____
_____
_____
_____
_____
_____
_____
_____
_____
_____
_____
_____
_____
_____
_____
_____
_____
_____
_____
_____
_____
_____

Has my food intake been sufficient in:

Protein ☐   Calcium ☐   Iron ☐   Omega 3 ☐   Vitamin C ☐   Fibre ☐

Notes

How has my mood been today?

_____

_____

_____

_____

_____

Is there anything I would do differently the following days?
(This could be in regard to your food intake, your discussions about
veganism with others, dealing with difficult scenarios with non-vegans
etc)

_____

_____

_____

_____

_____

_____

MY DAILY VEGAN DIARY

Day 145: _____

How did my day go?

_____
_____
_____
_____
_____
_____
_____
_____
_____
_____
_____
_____
_____
_____
_____
_____
_____
_____
_____
_____
_____
_____
_____
_____
_____
_____

Has my food intake been sufficient in:

Protein ☐   Calcium ☐   Iron ☐   Omega 3 ☐   Vitamin C ☐   Fibre ☐

Notes

How has my mood been today?

Is there anything I would do differently the following days?

(This could be in regard to your food intake, your discussions about veganism with others, dealing with difficult scenarios with non-vegans etc)

MY DAILY VEGAN DIARY

Day 146: _____

How did my day go?

_____
_____
_____
_____
_____
_____
_____
_____
_____
_____
_____
_____
_____
_____
_____
_____
_____
_____
_____
_____
_____
_____
_____
_____
_____
_____
_____

Has my food intake been sufficient in:

Protein ☐   Calcium ☐   Iron ☐   Omega 3 ☐   Vitamin C ☐   Fibre ☐

Notes

How has my mood been today?

_____

_____

_____

_____

_____

_____

Is there anything I would do differently the following days?

(This could be in regard to your food intake, your discussions about veganism with others, dealing with difficult scenarios with non-vegans etc)

_____

_____

_____

_____

_____

_____

_____

MY DAILY VEGAN DIARY

Day 147: _____

How did my day go?

_____
_____
_____
_____
_____
_____
_____
_____
_____
_____
_____
_____
_____
_____
_____
_____
_____
_____
_____
_____
_____
_____
_____
_____
_____
_____
_____
_____
_____

Has my food intake been sufficient in:

Protein ☐   Calcium ☐   Iron ☐   Omega 3 ☐   Vitamin C ☐   Fibre ☐

Notes

How has my mood been today?

_____
_____
_____
_____
_____
_____

Is there anything I would do differently the following days?
(This could be in regard to your food intake, your discussions about veganism with others, dealing with difficult scenarios with non-vegans etc)

_____
_____
_____
_____
_____
_____
_____

MY DAILY VEGAN DIARY

Day 148: _____

How did my day go?

_____
_____
_____
_____
_____
_____
_____
_____
_____
_____
_____
_____
_____
_____
_____
_____
_____
_____
_____
_____
_____
_____
_____
_____
_____
_____
_____
_____
_____
_____

Has my food intake been sufficient in:

Protein ☐   Calcium ☐   Iron ☐   Omega 3 ☐   Vitamin C ☐   Fibre ☐

Notes

How has my mood been today?

_____
_____
_____
_____
_____
_____

Is there anything I would do differently the following days?
(This could be in regard to your food intake, your discussions about
veganism with others, dealing with difficult scenarios with non-vegans
etc)

_____
_____
_____
_____
_____
_____
_____

MY DAILY VEGAN DIARY

Day 149.

How did my day go?

_____
_____
_____
_____
_____
_____
_____
_____
_____
_____
_____
_____
_____
_____
_____
_____
_____
_____
_____
_____
_____
_____
_____
_____
_____
_____
_____
_____

Has my food intake been sufficient in:

Protein ☐   Calcium ☐   Iron ☐   Omega 3 ☐   Vitamin C ☐   Fibre ☐

Notes

How has my mood been today?

_____
_____
_____
_____
_____
_____

Is there anything I would do differently the following days?

(This could be in regard to your food intake, your discussions about veganism with others, dealing with difficult scenarios with non-vegans etc)

_____
_____
_____
_____
_____
_____
_____

MY DAILY VEGAN DIARY

Day 150:

How did my day go?

_____
_____
_____
_____
_____
_____
_____
_____
_____
_____
_____
_____
_____
_____
_____
_____
_____
_____
_____
_____
_____
_____
_____
_____
_____
_____
_____
_____
_____

Has my food intake been sufficient in:

Protein ☐   Calcium ☐   Iron ☐   Omega 3 ☐   Vitamin C ☐   Fibre ☐

Notes

How has my mood been today?

_____

_____

_____

_____

_____

_____

Is there anything I would do differently the following days?
(This could be in regard to your food intake, your discussions about veganism with others, dealing with difficult scenarios with non-vegans etc)

_____

_____

_____

_____

_____

_____

_____

MY DAILY VEGAN DIARY

Day 151: _____

How did my day go?

_____
_____
_____
_____
_____
_____
_____
_____
_____
_____
_____
_____
_____
_____
_____
_____
_____
_____
_____
_____
_____
_____
_____
_____
_____
_____
_____
_____
_____

Has my food intake been sufficient in:

Protein ☐   Calcium ☐   Iron ☐   Omega 3 ☐   Vitamin C ☐   Fibre ☐

Notes

How has my mood been today?

_____
_____
_____
_____
_____
_____

Is there anything I would do differently the following days?
(This could be in regard to your food intake, your discussions about
veganism with others, dealing with difficult scenarios with non-vegans
etc)

_____
_____
_____
_____
_____
_____
_____

MY DAILY VEGAN DIARY

Day 152: _____

How did my day go?

_____
_____
_____
_____
_____
_____
_____
_____
_____
_____
_____
_____
_____
_____
_____
_____
_____
_____
_____
_____
_____
_____
_____
_____
_____
_____
_____
_____

Has my food intake been sufficient in:

Protein ☐   Calcium ☐   Iron ☐   Omega 3 ☐   Vitamin C ☐   Fibre ☐

Notes

How has my mood been today?

_____

_____

_____

_____

_____

_____

Is there anything I would do differently the following days?

(This could be in regard to your food intake, your discussions about veganism with others, dealing with difficult scenarios with non-vegans etc)

_____

_____

_____

_____

_____

_____

_____

MY DAILY VEGAN DIARY

Day 153.

How did my day go?

_____
_____
_____
_____
_____
_____
_____
_____
_____
_____
_____
_____
_____
_____
_____
_____
_____
_____
_____
_____
_____
_____
_____
_____
_____
_____
_____
_____

Has my food intake been sufficient in:

Protein ☐   Calcium ☐   Iron ☐   Omega 3 ☐   Vitamin C ☐   Fibre ☐

Notes

How has my mood been today?

_____

_____

_____

_____

_____

_____

Is there anything I would do differently the following days?

(This could be in regard to your food intake, your discussions about veganism with others, dealing with difficult scenarios with non-vegans etc)

_____

_____

_____

_____

_____

_____

_____

MY DAILY VEGAN DIARY

Day 154: _____

How did my day go?

_____
_____
_____
_____
_____
_____
_____
_____
_____
_____
_____
_____
_____
_____
_____
_____
_____
_____
_____
_____
_____
_____
_____
_____
_____
_____
_____
_____

Has my food intake been sufficient in:

Protein ☐   Calcium ☐   Iron ☐   Omega 3 ☐   Vitamin C ☐   Fibre ☐

Notes

How has my mood been today?

_____
_____
_____
_____
_____
_____

Is there anything I would do differently the following days?

(This could be in regard to your food intake, your discussions about veganism with others, dealing with difficult scenarios with non-vegans etc)

_____
_____
_____
_____
_____
_____
_____

MY DAILY VEGAN DIARY

Day 155: _____

How did my day go?

_____
_____
_____
_____
_____
_____
_____
_____
_____
_____
_____
_____
_____
_____
_____
_____
_____
_____
_____
_____
_____
_____
_____
_____
_____
_____
_____

Has my food intake been sufficient in:

Protein ☐   Calcium ☐   Iron ☐   Omega 3 ☐   Vitamin C ☐   Fibre ☐

Notes

How has my mood been today?

_____

_____

_____

_____

_____

_____

Is there anything I would do differently the following days?

(This could be in regard to your food intake, your discussions about veganism with others, dealing with difficult scenarios with non-vegans etc)

_____

_____

_____

_____

_____

_____

_____

MY DAILY VEGAN DIARY

Day 156: _____

How did my day go?

_____
_____
_____
_____
_____
_____
_____
_____
_____
_____
_____
_____
_____
_____
_____
_____
_____
_____
_____
_____
_____
_____
_____
_____
_____
_____

Has my food intake been sufficient in:

Protein ☐   Calcium ☐   Iron ☐   Omega 3 ☐   Vitamin C ☐   Fibre ☐

Notes

How has my mood been today?

_____
_____
_____
_____
_____
_____

Is there anything I would do differently the following days?
(This could be in regard to your food intake, your discussions about veganism with others, dealing with difficult scenarios with non-vegans etc)

_____
_____
_____
_____
_____
_____
_____

MY DAILY VEGAN DIARY

Day 157: _____

How did my day go?

_____
_____
_____
_____
_____
_____
_____
_____
_____
_____
_____
_____
_____
_____
_____
_____
_____
_____
_____
_____
_____
_____
_____
_____
_____
_____

Has my food intake been sufficient in:

Protein ☐   Calcium ☐   Iron ☐   Omega 3 ☐   Vitamin C ☐   Fibre ☐

Notes

How has my mood been today?

Is there anything I would do differently the following days?
(This could be in regard to your food intake, your discussions about
veganism with others, dealing with difficult scenarios with non-vegans
etc)

MY DAILY VEGAN DIARY

Day 158: _____

How did my day go?

_____

_____

_____

_____

_____

_____

_____

_____

_____

_____

_____

_____

_____

_____

_____

_____

_____

_____

_____

_____

_____

_____

_____

_____

_____

_____

_____

Has my food intake been sufficient in:

Protein ☐   Calcium ☐   Iron ☐   Omega 3 ☐   Vitamin C ☐   Fibre ☐

Notes

How has my mood been today?

Is there anything I would do differently the following days?

(This could be in regard to your food intake, your discussions about veganism with others, dealing with difficult scenarios with non-vegans etc)

MY DAILY VEGAN DIARY

Day 159: _____

How did my day go?

_____
_____
_____
_____
_____
_____
_____
_____
_____
_____
_____
_____
_____
_____
_____
_____
_____
_____
_____
_____
_____
_____
_____
_____
_____
_____
_____

Has my food intake been sufficient in:

Protein ☐   Calcium ☐   Iron ☐   Omega 3 ☐   Vitamin C ☐   Fibre ☐

Notes

How has my mood been today?

_____
_____
_____
_____
_____
_____

Is there anything I would do differently the following days?
(This could be in regard to your food intake, your discussions about veganism with others, dealing with difficult scenarios with non-vegans etc)

_____
_____
_____
_____
_____
_____
_____

MY DAILY VEGAN DIARY

Day 160. _____

How did my day go?

_____
_____
_____
_____
_____
_____
_____
_____
_____
_____
_____
_____
_____
_____
_____
_____
_____
_____
_____
_____
_____
_____
_____
_____
_____
_____
_____

Has my food intake been sufficient in:

Protein ☐   Calcium ☐   Iron ☐   Omega 3 ☐   Vitamin C ☐   Fibre ☐

Notes

How has my mood been today?

_____

_____

_____

_____

_____

_____

Is there anything I would do differently the following days?
(This could be in regard to your food intake, your discussions about veganism with others, dealing with difficult scenarios with non-vegans etc)

_____

_____

_____

_____

_____

_____

_____

MY DAILY VEGAN DIARY

Day 161: _____

How did my day go?

_____
_____
_____
_____
_____
_____
_____
_____
_____
_____
_____
_____
_____
_____
_____
_____
_____
_____
_____
_____
_____
_____
_____
_____
_____
_____
_____
_____

Has my food intake been sufficient in:

Protein ☐   Calcium ☐   Iron ☐   Omega 3 ☐   Vitamin C ☐   Fibre ☐

Notes

How has my mood been today?

Is there anything I would do differently the following days?
(This could be in regard to your food intake, your discussions about
veganism with others, dealing with difficult scenarios with non-vegans
etc)

MY DAILY VEGAN DIARY

Day 162: _____

How did my day go?

_____
_____
_____
_____
_____
_____
_____
_____
_____
_____
_____
_____
_____
_____
_____
_____
_____
_____
_____
_____
_____
_____
_____
_____
_____
_____
_____
_____
_____

Has my food intake been sufficient in:

Protein ☐   Calcium ☐   Iron ☐   Omega 3 ☐   Vitamin C ☐   Fibre ☐

Notes

How has my mood been today?

_____

_____

_____

_____

_____

_____

Is there anything I would do differently the following days?

(This could be in regard to your food intake, your discussions about veganism with others, dealing with difficult scenarios with non-vegans etc)

_____

_____

_____

_____

_____

_____

_____

MY DAILY VEGAN DIARY

Day 163.

How did my day go?

_____
_____
_____
_____
_____
_____
_____
_____
_____
_____
_____
_____
_____
_____
_____
_____
_____
_____
_____
_____
_____
_____
_____
_____
_____
_____
_____
_____

Has my food intake been sufficient in:

Protein ☐   Calcium ☐   Iron ☐   Omega 3 ☐   Vitamin C ☐   Fibre ☐

Notes

How has my mood been today?

_____

_____

_____

_____

_____

_____

Is there anything I would do differently the following days?

(This could be in regard to your food intake, your discussions about veganism with others, dealing with difficult scenarios with non-vegans etc)

_____

_____

_____

_____

_____

_____

_____

MY DAILY VEGAN DIARY

Day 164: _____

How did my day go?

_____
_____
_____
_____
_____
_____
_____
_____
_____
_____
_____
_____
_____
_____
_____
_____
_____
_____
_____
_____
_____
_____
_____
_____
_____
_____
_____

Has my food intake been sufficient in:

Protein ☐   Calcium ☐   Iron ☐   Omega 3 ☐   Vitamin C ☐   Fibre ☐

Notes

How has my mood been today?

_____

_____

_____

_____

_____

_____

Is there anything I would do differently the following days?

(This could be in regard to your food intake, your discussions about

veganism with others, dealing with difficult scenarios with non-vegans

etc)

_____

_____

_____

_____

_____

_____

_____

MY DAILY VEGAN DIARY

Day 165: _____

How did my day go?

_____
_____
_____
_____
_____
_____
_____
_____
_____
_____
_____
_____
_____
_____
_____
_____
_____
_____
_____
_____
_____
_____
_____
_____
_____
_____
_____

Has my food intake been sufficient in:

Protein ☐   Calcium ☐   Iron ☐   Omega 3 ☐   Vitamin C ☐   Fibre ☐

Notes

How has my mood been today?

_____

_____

_____

_____

_____

_____

Is there anything I would do differently the following days?

(This could be in regard to your food intake, your discussions about

veganism with others, dealing with difficult scenarios with non-vegans

etc)

_____

_____

_____

_____

_____

_____

_____

MY DAILY VEGAN DIARY

Day 166: _____

How did my day go?

_____
_____
_____
_____
_____
_____
_____
_____
_____
_____
_____
_____
_____
_____
_____
_____
_____
_____
_____
_____
_____
_____
_____
_____
_____
_____
_____

Has my food intake been sufficient in:

Protein ☐   Calcium ☐   Iron ☐   Omega 3 ☐   Vitamin C ☐   Fibre ☐

Notes

How has my mood been today?

_____

_____

_____

_____

_____

_____

Is there anything I would do differently the following days?

(This could be in regard to your food intake, your discussions about

veganism with others, dealing with difficult scenarios with non-vegans

etc)

_____

_____

_____

_____

_____

_____

_____

MY DAILY VEGAN DIARY

Day 167: _____

How did my day go?

_____
_____
_____
_____
_____
_____
_____
_____
_____
_____
_____
_____
_____
_____
_____
_____
_____
_____
_____
_____
_____
_____
_____
_____
_____
_____
_____
_____
_____

Has my food intake been sufficient in:

Protein ☐   Calcium ☐   Iron ☐   Omega 3 ☐ Vitamin C ☐ Fibre ☐

Notes

How has my mood been today?

_____

_____

_____

_____

_____

_____

Is there anything I would do differently the following days?
(This could be in regard to your food intake, your discussions about veganism with others, dealing with difficult scenarios with non-vegans etc)

_____

_____

_____

_____

_____

_____

_____

MY DAILY VEGAN DIARY

Day 168: _____

How did my day go?

_____
_____
_____
_____
_____
_____
_____
_____
_____
_____
_____
_____
_____
_____
_____
_____
_____
_____
_____
_____
_____
_____
_____
_____
_____
_____
_____

Has my food intake been sufficient in:

Protein ☐   Calcium ☐   Iron ☐   Omega 3 ☐   Vitamin C ☐   Fibre ☐

Notes

How has my mood been today?

_____
_____
_____
_____
_____
_____

Is there anything I would do differently the following days?

(This could be in regard to your food intake, your discussions about veganism with others, dealing with difficult scenarios with non-vegans etc)

_____
_____
_____
_____
_____
_____
_____

MY DAILY VEGAN DIARY

Day 169.

How did my day go?

_____

_____

_____

_____

_____

_____

_____

_____

_____

_____

_____

_____

_____

_____

_____

_____

_____

_____

_____

_____

_____

_____

_____

_____

_____

_____

_____

_____

Has my food intake been sufficient in:

Protein ☐   Calcium ☐   Iron ☐   Omega 3 ☐   Vitamin C ☐   Fibre ☐

Notes

How has my mood been today?

_____

_____

_____

_____

_____

_____

Is there anything I would do differently the following days?

(This could be in regard to your food intake, your discussions about veganism with others, dealing with difficult scenarios with non-vegans etc)

_____

_____

_____

_____

_____

_____

_____

MY DAILY VEGAN DIARY

Day 170: _____

How did my day go?

_____
_____
_____
_____
_____
_____
_____
_____
_____
_____
_____
_____
_____
_____
_____
_____
_____
_____
_____
_____
_____
_____
_____
_____
_____
_____
_____

Has my food intake been sufficient in:

Protein ☐   Calcium ☐   Iron ☐   Omega 3 ☐   Vitamin C ☐   Fibre ☐

Notes

How has my mood been today?

_____

_____

_____

_____

_____

_____

Is there anything I would do differently the following days?
(This could be in regard to your food intake, your discussions about
veganism with others, dealing with difficult scenarios with non-vegans
etc)

_____

_____

_____

_____

_____

_____

_____

MY DAILY VEGAN DIARY

Day 171:

How did my day go?

_____
_____
_____
_____
_____
_____
_____
_____
_____
_____
_____
_____
_____
_____
_____
_____
_____
_____
_____
_____
_____
_____
_____
_____
_____
_____
_____
_____
_____

Has my food intake been sufficient in:

Protein ☐   Calcium ☐   Iron ☐   Omega 3 ☐   Vitamin C ☐   Fibre ☐

Notes

How has my mood been today?

Is there anything I would do differently the following days?
(This could be in regard to your food intake, your discussions about
veganism with others, dealing with difficult scenarios with non-vegans
etc)

MY DAILY VEGAN DIARY

Day 172: _____

How did my day go?

_____
_____
_____
_____
_____
_____
_____
_____
_____
_____
_____
_____
_____
_____
_____
_____
_____
_____
_____
_____
_____
_____
_____
_____
_____
_____

Has my food intake been sufficient in:

Protein ☐   Calcium ☐   Iron ☐   Omega 3 ☐   Vitamin C ☐   Fibre ☐

Notes

How has my mood been today?

_____

_____

_____

_____

_____

_____

Is there anything I would do differently the following days?
(This could be in regard to your food intake, your discussions about veganism with others, dealing with difficult scenarios with non-vegans etc)

_____

_____

_____

_____

_____

_____

_____

MY DAILY VEGAN DIARY

Day 173: _____

How did my day go?

_____
_____
_____
_____
_____
_____
_____
_____
_____
_____
_____
_____
_____
_____
_____
_____
_____
_____
_____
_____
_____
_____
_____
_____
_____
_____
_____
_____
_____

Has my food intake been sufficient in:

Protein ☐   Calcium ☐   Iron ☐   Omega 3 ☐   Vitamin C ☐   Fibre ☐

Notes

How has my mood been today?

_____

_____

_____

_____

_____

_____

Is there anything I would do differently the following days?

(This could be in regard to your food intake, your discussions about veganism with others, dealing with difficult scenarios with non-vegans etc)

_____

_____

_____

_____

_____

_____

MY DAILY VEGAN DIARY

Day 174:

How did my day go?

_____
_____
_____
_____
_____
_____
_____
_____
_____
_____
_____
_____
_____
_____
_____
_____
_____
_____
_____
_____
_____
_____
_____
_____
_____
_____
_____

Has my food intake been sufficient in:

Protein ☐   Calcium ☐   Iron ☐   Omega 3 ☐   Vitamin C ☐   Fibre ☐

Notes

How has my mood been today?

Is there anything I would do differently the following days?
(This could be in regard to your food intake, your discussions about
veganism with others, dealing with difficult scenarios with non-vegans
etc)

MY DAILY VEGAN DIARY

Day 175: _____

How did my day go?

_____
_____
_____
_____
_____
_____
_____
_____
_____
_____
_____
_____
_____
_____
_____
_____
_____
_____
_____
_____
_____
_____
_____
_____
_____
_____
_____

Has my food intake been sufficient in:

Protein ☐   Calcium ☐   Iron ☐   Omega 3 ☐   Vitamin C ☐   Fibre ☐

Notes

How has my mood been today?

_____
_____
_____
_____
_____
_____

Is there anything I would do differently the following days?

(This could be in regard to your food intake, your discussions about

veganism with others, dealing with difficult scenarios with non-vegans

etc)

_____
_____
_____
_____
_____
_____
_____

MY DAILY VEGAN DIARY

Day 176: _____

How did my day go?

_____

_____

_____

_____

_____

_____

_____

_____

_____

_____

_____

_____

_____

_____

_____

_____

_____

_____

_____

_____

_____

_____

_____

_____

_____

_____

_____

_____

_____

Has my food intake been sufficient in:

Protein ☐   Calcium ☐   Iron ☐   Omega 3 ☐   Vitamin C ☐   Fibre ☐

Notes

How has my mood been today?

_____

_____

_____

_____

_____

_____

Is there anything I would do differently the following days?

(This could be in regard to your food intake, your discussions about veganism with others, dealing with difficult scenarios with non-vegans etc)

_____

_____

_____

_____

_____

_____

_____

MY DAILY VEGAN DIARY

Day 177: _____

How did my day go?

_____
_____
_____
_____
_____
_____
_____
_____
_____
_____
_____
_____
_____
_____
_____
_____
_____
_____
_____
_____
_____
_____
_____
_____
_____
_____
_____
_____
_____

Has my food intake been sufficient in:

Protein ☐   Calcium ☐   Iron ☐   Omega 3 ☐   Vitamin C ☐   Fibre ☐

Notes

How has my mood been today?

_____
_____
_____
_____
_____
_____

Is there anything I would do differently the following days?

(This could be in regard to your food intake, your discussions about veganism with others, dealing with difficult scenarios with non-vegans etc)

_____
_____
_____
_____
_____
_____
_____

MY DAILY VEGAN DIARY

Day 178: _____

How did my day go?

_____
_____
_____
_____
_____
_____
_____
_____
_____
_____
_____
_____
_____
_____
_____
_____
_____
_____
_____
_____
_____
_____
_____
_____
_____
_____
_____
_____
_____

Has my food intake been sufficient in:

Protein ☐   Calcium ☐   Iron ☐   Omega 3 ☐   Vitamin C ☐   Fibre ☐

Notes

How has my mood been today?

_____

_____

_____

_____

_____

_____

Is there anything I would do differently the following days?

(This could be in regard to your food intake, your discussions about

veganism with others, dealing with difficult scenarios with non-vegans

etc)

_____

_____

_____

_____

_____

_____

_____

MY DAILY VEGAN DIARY

Day 179: _____

How did my day go?

_____
_____
_____
_____
_____
_____
_____
_____
_____
_____
_____
_____
_____
_____
_____
_____
_____
_____
_____
_____
_____
_____
_____
_____
_____
_____
_____

Has my food intake been sufficient in:

Protein ☐   Calcium ☐   Iron ☐   Omega 3 ☐   Vitamin C ☐   Fibre ☐

Notes

How has my mood been today?

_____

_____

_____

_____

_____

_____

Is there anything I would do differently the following days?

(This could be in regard to your food intake, your discussions about veganism with others, dealing with difficult scenarios with non-vegans etc)

_____

_____

_____

_____

_____

_____

MY DAILY VEGAN DIARY

Day 180: _____

How did my day go?

_____
_____
_____
_____
_____
_____
_____
_____
_____
_____
_____
_____
_____
_____
_____
_____
_____
_____
_____
_____
_____
_____
_____
_____
_____
_____

Has my food intake been sufficient in:

Protein ☐   Calcium ☐   Iron ☐   Omega 3 ☐   Vitamin C ☐   Fibre ☐

Notes

How has my mood been today?

_____

_____

_____

_____

_____

_____

Is there anything I would do differently the following days?

(This could be in regard to your food intake, your discussions about veganism with others, dealing with difficult scenarios with non-vegans etc)

_____

_____

_____

_____

_____

_____

_____

MY DAILY VEGAN DIARY

Day 181:

How did my day go?

_____
_____
_____
_____
_____
_____
_____
_____
_____
_____
_____
_____
_____
_____
_____
_____
_____
_____
_____
_____
_____
_____
_____
_____
_____
_____

Has my food intake been sufficient in:

Protein ☐   Calcium ☐   Iron ☐   Omega 3 ☐   Vitamin C ☐   Fibre ☐

Notes

How has my mood been today?

_____

_____

_____

_____

_____

_____

Is there anything I would do differently the following days?

(This could be in regard to your food intake, your discussions about veganism with others, dealing with difficult scenarios with non-vegans etc)

_____

_____

_____

_____

_____

_____

_____

CONGRATULATIONS

Day 182: 6 months a vegan (or 6 months monitoring
your thoughts as a vegan)

How do you feel today? What can you see that has changed and developed
in your life journey as a vegan?

_____
_____
_____
_____
_____
_____
_____
_____
_____
_____
_____
_____
_____
_____
_____
_____
_____
_____
_____
_____
_____
_____
_____

SUGGESTED READING

-Veganuary

A great little book and plenty of resources if you join online.

-Vistopia

Clare Mann – This is a brilliant book in regard to the psychological

well-being of new vegans; a must read book!

-Why we love dogs, eat pigs and wear cows

Dr Melanie Joy (Vegan psychology) A must read

- Beyond Beliefs

Dr Melanie Joy (well-being, psychology and relationships) significant read

- The World Peace Diet

Will Tuttle (vegan philosophy) Beautiful book

- The China Study

Colin T Campbell (research) Fascinating and informative

- Vegan Savvy

Azmina Govindji (Nutrition made simple) Great for those wanting to be

extra careful with a healthy wholefood diet.

SUGGESTED YOUTUBE CHANNELS

- Plant-based news

(Interesting news articles and information, progress stories)

- Mic the Vegan

(Diet research with humour)

- Live Kindly

(Interesting news articles and information, progress stories)

- Nutritional Facts - Dr Greger

(Dietary research updates)

- The Physician's Committee

(Health and vegan/plant-based diet science)

- Earthling Ed

Animal Activism and education

- Joey Carbstrong

Animal Activist

CHARITIES SUPPORTING ANIMALS & VEGAN ORGANIZATIONS

- Animal Aid

- Animal Equality

- Humane Society International

- Peta

- Surge

- Viva

- Vegan Society

REFERENCES TO NUTRITION INFORMATION FOR SUPPLEMENTS

- Nutritionfacts.org

- Dr Greger (website) How Not to Die (book)

- Vitamins and Minerals — Sara Rose (book)

- National Health Service website - UK

MEALS TO VEGANIZE

Think of any meaty or dairy based meals that you would like to veganize — write a list and then you can research online recipes

_____
_____
_____
_____
_____
_____
_____
_____
_____
_____
_____
_____
_____
_____
_____
_____
_____
_____
_____
_____
_____
_____
_____
_____

NOTES

Any tips or reminders for yourself

_____
_____
_____
_____
_____
_____
_____
_____
_____
_____
_____
_____
_____
_____
_____
_____
_____
_____
_____
_____
_____
_____
_____
_____

Wishing you well on your journey towards making a difference to the animals, the environment and your own health and well-being.

Eat with love in your heart and mind so you feed and nourish your body and soul....

May all beings be happy and free!

Love, peace and Light....

Kasarah Vegan xx

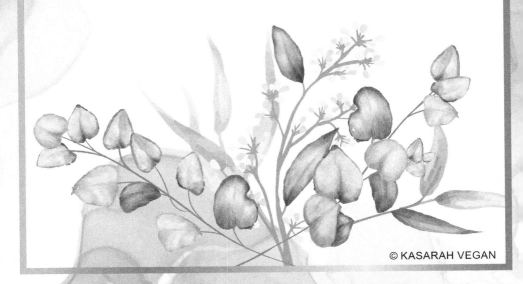

Printed in Great Britain
by Amazon